Dedicated to my family.

Acknowledgements

I wish to thank my daughter, Susan Lee Reardon, for turning my odd hen-scratches into beautiful illustrations.

I also wish to thank Paul Salsbury for driving me to odd locations at odd times in order to take photos

Thanks also to the sustainable farmers I interviewed: Asher and Wendy Burkhart-Spiegel of Common Thread, info@ commonthreadcsa.com and Sarah Huftalen of Huftalen Farms, Huftalenfarms@aol.com. Also, thanks to Melissa Shupp of the CNY Green Bucket Project.

Appreciation goes to all those church members, family members and friends who submitted recipes and photos for Chapter 12. Some of the proceeds will benefit the Climate Action Sub-committee of the Unitarian Universalist Church of Utica which gave me the idea and incentive to write this book.

Thanks also to Michael Weir and Patricia Evans for help with editing.

Sally West Carman

Contents

Introduction

Part One
The Science of Climate

Food

Part Two
Food Production

Chapter three
A little dirt is good for you 26

Chapter four
Corny is no joke 34

Chapter five
What's the beef? 40

Chapter six
Something is fishy

Chapter seven
Water, water everywhere, but not a drop to drink

Chapter eight
A tree grows in your backyard

Part Three
Buying and storing food

Chapter nine
Keep Mother Nature on your side

Food

Food

Sally West Carman

Introduction

Food

Foreword

"We stand now where two roads diverge. But unlike the roads in <u>Robert Frost</u>'s familiar poem, they are not equally fair. The road we have long been traveling is deceptively easy, a smooth superhighway on which we progress with great speed, but at its end lies disaster. The other fork of the road — the one less traveled by — offers our last, our only chance to reach a destination that assures the preservation of the earth."

-Rachel Carson, <u>Silent Spring</u>

Concern for the environment tugs strongly at my heart. I think it is because of a desire for a better future for my children grandchildren and great-grandchildren. Also, as I grow older, continuing to live with good health becomes increasingly important.

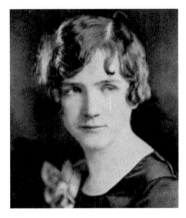

Rachel Carson, photo courtesy of Wikipedia.

I was impacted by *Silent Spring* written by Rachel Carson in the '60s, and *Diet for a Small Planet* by Frances Moore Lappé in the '70s. This concern translates into a compulsion to do something, some might say a spiritual feeling. Concern for the impact that food has on the environment and consequently climate change is a natural progression.

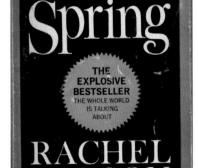

Food and water are so basic to life, necessary for human existence to continue. Food impacts our health in so many ways. Food is also something largely under our control. We choose what we put into our bodies each day. Many things of which we are not consciously aware can have a major impact on climate change.

Therefore, this book was born, spawned by meetings of members of the Climate Change Sub-committee of the Unitarian Universalist Church of Utica. Many of the recipes included have been tested and enjoyed by members of the congregation. Facts have been gleaned from scientific studies I have researched. All sources have been credited in the endnotes and the bibliography.

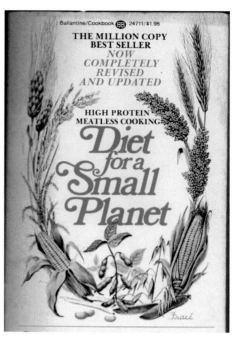

My worn copy of Frances Moore Lappe's book.

Since obtaining my Master of Arts Degree in Human Nutrition from Syracuse University in 1982, I have had a dream of applying that knowledge to a book about good nutrition. Coupling this with a concern about the rapidly changing climate became an incentive to get started.

When I worked briefly as a dietitian, I learned very early that people do not like to be told what to eat, and seldom listen to advice. However, I will make yet another attempt to influence food choices. At least in a book, no one can talk back to me, at least not immediately.

Our hope is that this book will "light your fire" about all that we can do to make the world a better place, and slow the impact of climate change. We know this is an elusive goal, but we hope to make at least a small difference.

Introduction

Earth provides enough to satisfy every man's needs, but not every man's greed.

-Mahatma Gandhi

As much as one-half of climate change can be traced to our food and drink. What we put in our mouths is something that each of us can easily control. If we care about our health, we **must** be concerned. If we care about our planet, we **must** be concerned and it is **time** to take action.

The mission of this book is to bring together some of the up-to-date scientific thought about the relationship of food and drink to good health and to environmental quality. It does not rely on original research. Instead it hopes to summarize some of the current thinking on the topic in an understandable manner. Many sources have been studied to include factual information.

Using many visuals and some humor, we hope to bring some light to a dark subject. By presenting this in easy-to-digest bites, we hope to contradict some of the sound bites presented by the media. The media has a tendency to over-simplify and exaggerate scientific studies that have not been fully veted. Also, the power of corporations and advertisers to sway the facts to suit the purposes of the almighty dollar is ever-present.

Follow the money

Much of the information we read on-line and in newspapers, or see on TV, or hear on the radio has been tainted. Major interests are using money to slant the news in a direction most profitable to them. Oil companies foster climate change deniers and thwart

Food

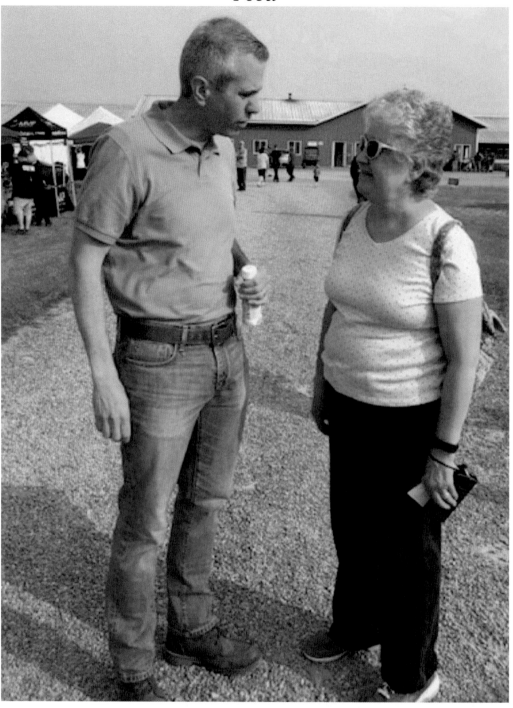

At a local farm open house I had an opportunity to discuss climate change with my local district congressman, Representative Anthony Brindisi. Though he may not agree with all my views, he was willing to listen.

the development of alternative energy because they are in the business of making money through oil. Chemical companies like Monsanto (now owned by Bayer) say that their products are necessary to produce more food.

The direction has become very political. Michael Mann, a Pennsylvania State professor and author of the "hockey stick" graph demonstrating global warming, has even received death threats. Other scientists are shamed and criticized for presenting their research results.

Now is the time for action

Climate change is such a complex and far-reaching subject, with significant consequences for the future of human life. The world is whirling and changing so quickly that we have to hang on in order to prevent "falling off." The health of our children and grandchildren hangs in the balance.

The good news is that our diet is something that we can impact in a positive way. The road to less heart disease, diabetes and obesity is the path we wish to follow, and hope that you do as well.

Everyone get discouraged because the problem seems so large. However, there are things that each of us can do individually. If enough people live in environmentally sensitive ways, the impact can be huge.

This book is based on evidence from science and scientists, as noted by the extensive endnotes. You may want to think of each chapter as a separate essay, and read in whatever order you wish. Perhaps you will skip over parts you already know. Or you may use this as a reference to look up information.

My wish is for you to live a long and healthy life, and your family as well. Please read on.

Food

Part One
The Science of Climate

Food

Chapter one

There is a unity to all things in the universe
and the light of the spirit shines in all things.
Each action taken, each thought conceived, affects all else
and, thus we are all co-creators of the reality around us.

May we therefore, with conscious recognition and humility,
understand that our choices in how to grow
and consume the food we need to live will,
for better or worse, affect the earth, our interdependent web of life,
and the universe in which we live.

Jay Hagenbuch

Go for the goal?

Usually we strive to reach a goal, whether to ring the bell at the top of the column at the carnival, or the football championship, or the college scholarship. However, we have reached a new goal that we were not aiming to achieve.

In May 2019 the peak of carbon dioxide in our atmosphere reached a record amount of 414.8 parts per million (ppm). This doesn't mean anything to us until we find out that it is the highest level in the history of humans on this earth, and may be the highest in three million years. (1) Though levels are usually the highest in May, this is a sign that not enough is being done to control these rising levels.

You may ask how we know the history of the earth so far in the past. This is determined by scientists by measuring carbon in ice-core samples in the far north. Using powered drills, cores are obtained as much as two miles below the surface, which are as old as 800,000 years. Tiny bubbles in the ice are used to measure carbon dioxide in the atmosphere at that time. (2)

Food

Since 1958, measurements of the level of carbon dioxide in the atmosphere has been measured at the Mauna Loa Observatory in Hawaii run by the Scripps Institution of Oceanography of San Diego, California. This continual increase is known as the Keeling Curve, named after Charles Keeling, who began making the first observations. His son, Ralph Keeling, now directs the programs at Scripps. (3)

Why should we care?

Political opinions sometimes dispute the impact of humans on climate change. Some say it is due to cyclical changes. However, the vast majority of scientists agree that much of climate change is due to human interaction with the environment. The changes we are seeing are much greater than would be predicted by natural phenomenon and the usual cyclical changes in weather. A report of the Intergovernmental Panel on Climate Change (IPCC) released in 2018 gave scientific evidence that these massive changes that we are experiencing result primarily from human interaction. (4)

You can't lick a hockey stick

The fact that the climate is changing is indisputable. Charts demonstrate the steady rise in air temperature. A chart developed by Michael Mann, Distinguished Professor of Meteorology at Pennsylvania State University, demonstrates the

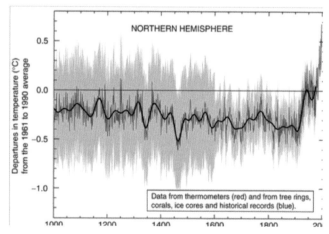

This graph was developed by Michael Mann in 1999 and has been the standard to illustrate the increase in global warming using many different measurements. https://green.blogs.nytimes. com/2010/09/23/the-hockey-stick-lives/

precipitous rise in average temperature which looks more like a hockey stick than a scientific chart. (5)

Many other studies have shown that the temperature is rising. (6) Much of this is attributed to the burning of fossil fuels.

Weather events are becoming more severe each year: massive wildfires in California, drought in the Midwest, flooding in the South and Northeast, and an increasing number of tornadoes in the South and Midwest.

Build your ark now

The measures of ocean depth show that water is rising. Photos of glaciers show that the giant glaciers of the most northern and southern continents are like huge melting popsicles.

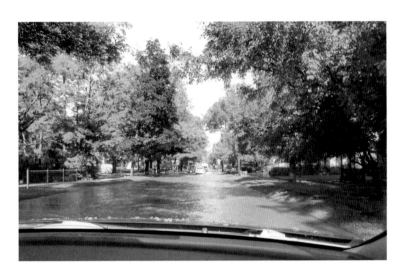

A scene of flooding in my neighborhood in 2018, and we are not near a large body of water.

Polar bears are jumping over widening gaps in the ice. Penguins look like a video game, falling into the frigid northern water. Antarctica, Iceland and Greenland are losing land because of increasing sea temperature.

Some areas such as the Northeast U.S. and Great Britain are experiencing increased rain. Floods have become more common. This is causing increasing amounts of property damage as named hurricanes use up all the letters of the alphabet in finding new nomenclature.

The East Coast of the U.S. has been inundated by too much water and major flooding. Hurricane Sandy in 2012, dubbed Frankenstorm by the National Weather Service, caused large parts of the famous Jersey Shore to be washed away and much of

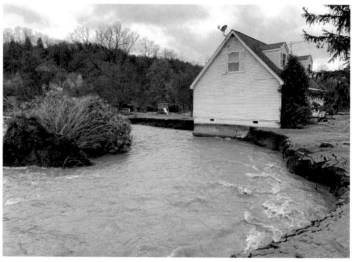

Halloween night 2019 caused massive flooding in our area. I had two sump pumps running though I am not near a creek. This house lost much of its foundation. Before that night, the creek was not even visible from the house and the owner did not have flood insurance. Photo courtesy of Glenn Coin, Syracuse Post-Standard.

Staten Island to be underwater. It caused $71 billion in economic damage and damaged or destroyed 650,000 homes and 72 lives were lost. (My daughter and family were forced to rebuilt their house on the shore.) Even the New York Stock Exchange was forced to close for the first time in 27 years. (7)

Also, Hurricane Katrina in 2005 that devastated New Orleans has been deemed another one of the worst storms, costing $108 billion to $250 billion. It left 1,836 people dead. (8) Hurricane Harvey hit Texas in August 2017 and was considered second in this Hall of Fame of famous storms. Harvey cost $25.5 billion. (9)

Manhattan is currently building steel barriers to protect its underground subways. The Naval Base in Norfolk, Virginia has been continually flooded, causing a national security threat. It has suffered nine floods in the last ten years. (10) (More in Chapter Seven.)

And the storms continue.

Permafrost is not permanent

Since it is far north of most of us, we do not think about the so-called permafrost which "comprises 24% of the land of the Northern Hemisphere." (11) Permafrost was called that because it was considered a permanent layer of frozen water in the far north. However, because of *particularly hot summers in 1998, 2010, 2011 and 2012* the top layer of permafrost began to melt. Recently the permafrost has actually caught on fire. (12)

Why does this concern us? Because as the permafrost thaws, *it can release large portions of carbon dioxide and methane, gases that contribute to the greenhouse effect.* (13)   It also changes the composition of plant life that can survive. Unfortunately, it appears that the permafrost is melting at a rate greater than had been anticipated.

This also means that more water is released, raising the level of the oceans. Since 40% of the population of the U.S. lives near water, the possibility of a gigantic problem is obvious.

Even famous sand beaches exist because giant cranes scoop up the sand that has washed out to sea. These claws deposit sand back on land again, in a futile attempt to hold back Mother Nature.

Water here, water there, not in the right places

On the other hand, in other areas around the world, lack of water is presenting a new crisis situation. In Cape Town, South Africa, water rationing had become the new norm. In the Midwest plains of the U.S., dry land is approaching the Dust Bowl stage so eloquently described in *The Grapes of Wrath* by John Steinbeck that was published in 1939. (14) The sand storms in 1930s forced many to move farther west. Again, drought is plaguing the Midwest and West. (15)

Food

You can't fool Mother Nature

The West Coast of the U.S. has seen unprecedented weather events. First there were the forest fires that destroyed even the homes of the rich and famous. These were followed by homes being swallowed by giant mud slides because the mountains and hills had been denuded by the fires.

A wildfire in 2018 in California named the Camp Fire destroyed an entire town with the misnomer of Paradise. These fires spread so quickly there was no time for evacuation.

If this were not enough, water emergencies have forced some people to turn off their taps and not water their lawns. Tributaries of water such as the Colorado River which supplies water to many western states continue to get more and more narrow.

Much of the nation depends of the crops that California produces or that come from Chile and other South American countries. Those of us in the East are supplied with seasonal produce year-round, even though it travels many miles. We can have almonds and lettuce for our salads, grapes (and a lot of high-quality wine), strawberries, tomatoes, walnuts and surprisingly, hay at any time of year.

Some family farms such as the Lundberg Family Farms in California are using sustainable methods of agriculture and are starting to cultivate quinoa in the United States. (16) Common Thread, a C.S.A. in Madison, New York has developed some intriguing new methods. (See Chapter nine)

The Grey Rock Farm in Central New York is using transitional methods to produce a variety of food products. (17) Some entrepreneurs are even producing tomatoes in the winter using greenhouses.

The rest of the winter crop comes from Florida and the South. Much of our citrus fruit originates there. Those states have also been devastated by major storms. Not to mention the giant sink holes that have been developing in Florida, a state that is floating like a raft on a system of underground water-filled caves. (18) As more people retire and migrate there, it is sinking more as water use grows exponentially. Everyone wants to live on water, but no one can live underwater for very long.

Large parts of the United States exist on fault lines. We never know when one of these will open up and cause untold disaster. An earthquake was recently felt in Mexico City, another in the Caribbean.

Better known as hydro-fracking, companies add to the earthquake danger by drilling deep in the earth and sending down billions of gallons of water to retrieve natural gas. Multiple earthquakes in Oklahoma have demonstrated this problem. "The Oklahoma Geological Survey has determined that the majority of recent earthquakes in central and north-central Oklahoma are very likely triggered by the injection of produced water in disposal wells." (19)

There may not be any more storms each year in terms of numbers, but they have been much more virulent. We are constantly fighting nature. (20) Instead of living by nature's rules, we think we can overcome the odds, only to find that nature often wins again. We are continually proving that *You can't fool Mother Nature.*

Roots of terrorism

In many cases poverty, hunger and the lack of clean drinking water can lead to insurrection and war. People who are poor and people who are hungry fight for a better life. Lack of food and water causes people to get desperate. If their neighbors have a lot more, they want some of the action. Unscrupulous leaders use this to their own advantage to stir up trouble and get more for themselves in the process. The terrible crisis in Syria and the strife in the Sudan are a few examples.

Food

According retired General David Titley in an interview by Christiana Amanpour on PBS, the drought in Syria was a causative factor for the long-term war. (21) The leaders decided to grow barley with huge irrigation projects that were successful for a while. However, when water ran out and the crops failed, the people were unemployed and hungry. They were desperate and ripe for ISIS propaganda.

Water and the lack of it may become the most destabilizing force in the future.

Get your oxygen mask now

The air we breathe is essential to human life. Photos of people in the capital of China wearing masks to walk to work is one example. The smog in Los Angeles is another. Greenhouse gases are not only causing the temperature to climb, but the particulates in the air threaten the very air we breathe.

What are greenhouse gases? The most publicized one is an increase in carbon dioxide (CO_2). However, methane, though in smaller quantities, has a much greater effect. A group called the Carbon Dioxide Coalition is attempting to distort the facts by touting the benefits of CO_2. It is true that CO_2 is necessary for the growth of plants and trees. However, too much of a good thing forms a layer around the earth, trapping excess heat and radiation from the sun.

No laughing matter

Nitrous oxide is another greenhouse gas and is considered third on the list of problem gases. Otherwise known as "laughing gas", it is commonly used by dentists for sedation. It is also used in spray cans such as for whipped cream and oil. According to studies presented by the National Institute of Health, it is responsible for about five percent of the global greenhouse gas effect. (22)

Oil, gas and coal are disappearing

Despite heroic and land-destroying attempts to find more oil deposits, we are not making any more oil and thus it is a disappearing resource. Despite hydro-fracking using monumental amounts of water and huge drilling rigs, disrupting the geography of the land, we are not making more natural gas. Coal mines are being depleted and cause a huge loss of miners' lives, as has occurred in China. Oil, gas and coal were formed by pressure of the earth during millenniums of time. Humans are **not capable** of manufacturing any more of these natural resources. They have a diminishing limit which will be reached by our grandchildren and great-grandchildren.

There is hope

All this gloom and doom may cause us to despair and give up. However, there is much we as individuals and collectively in groups can do. The following pages will show what is being done and what can be done to take the "path less traveled." We can plant trees. We can support farmers who are returning to the old methods. We can grow our own food. We can buy local and buy organic foods. We can avoid processed foods. We can limit waste by reusing and recycling. Our votes count when we support politicians who care about these issues. (23)

Three evil elements that are contributing to climate change are carbon dioxide, which is the largest in amount, methane, which is a lesser amount but much more potent, and nitrous oxide to a lesser degree.

Food

Chapter two
Our Chemical Bath

Why should we tolerate a diet of weak poisons, a home in insipid surroundings, a circle of acquaintances who are not quite our enemies, the noise of motors with just enough relief to prevent insanity? Who would want to live in a world which is just not quite fatal?"
-Rachel Carson, Silent Spring

Unintended consequences

In 1971 Rachel Carson in her book *The Silent Spring* launched an attack on the widespread use of DDT (dichloro-diphenyl-trichloroethane), which was used to kill insects following World War II. It was used to rapidly kill mosquitoes which spread malaria, thus was considered a blessing.

However, in 1972 DDT was banned in the United States after the EPA (Environmental Protection Agency) found that it was a probable human carcinogen (cause of cancer). Sadly, those of us born before 1972 still carry DDT in our blood. (Watch where you spread your ashes.) (1)

An even greater menace is the use of glyphosate, the main component of Roundup manufactured by Monsanto. It is used for controlling weeds on commercial farms, golf courses and home lawns. The invention of GMOs allowed that chemical to be used on crops thus increasing yields.

A deal with the devil

Ironically enough, it was a Jewish chemist, Fritz Haber, who developed a method to synthesize nitrogen. According to Josh

Food

Tickell in his book *Kiss the Ground*, Haber worked with Carl Bosch to refine the design, and they founded the Haber-Bosch Plant to produce ammonium nitrate for fertilizer use. At about the same time Germany was heading toward World War I and enlisted the company to make nitrogen for bombs. (2)

The great antithesis - more food for people to live and more bombs for them to die.

An unintended consequence was that the synthetic nitrogen also was loved by weeds, and these attracted various pests. Haber then found a way to make pesticides to kill the pests and weeds. These became the basis for poison gas used as a nerve agent to kill soldiers in a horrible way during World War I. Later Fritz Haber was forced to flee Germany when that gas was used to exterminate the Jewish people during the Holocaust of World War II. (3)

Beware of unintended consequences.

A chemical bath

An invention in the 1970s was a new chemical to control weeds, glyphosate (N-phosphonomethol glycine) developed after World War II. It works by shutting down plant growth and is better known as RoundUp. The California DPA calls it carcinogenic. It is routinely sprayed on crops before harvest, mostly on corn and soy that are GMOs designed to resist the chemical (4)

However, the unintended consequences are that the weeds become more and more resistant to this chemical necessitating more to be used. Then it creeps into our food supply. The International Agency for Research on Cancer's 2015 report classified glyphosate as a "probable human carcinogen." (5)

Another similar chemical is called **atrazine** and has been banned by the European Union. It disturbs human hormones and is the most common herbicide found in U.S. groundwater according to the U.S. Geological Survey. (6). It can lead to lower mental development and poorer attention spans. (See Center for the Health Assessment of Mothers and Children, a joint project with the University of California at Berkeley). (7)

Also, the manufacturers of larger and increasingly more expensive farm equipment are making it more expensive to farm on a small scale. Large chemical manufacturers have a financial interest in the increased use of fertilizers. Seed companies get involved too, as more Genetically Modified Organisms (GMOs) seeds are being used. Banks find it easier to lend to the large producers so that they can roll in a larger profit. (8)

The chemical herbicides become less effective as the weeds modify and are stronger than the weed killers. (6) They are survivors, and if they had mouths, they could laugh at those chemical makers.

Glyphosate the principal chemical found in Round-Up is now being used so extensively that it is showing up in our food. Oats and products made from oats are found to have this chemical, albeit in small amounts. However, small amounts build up. Some of those oal cereals we feed to our babies are so easy and inexpensive. But younger and smaller bodies are more sensitive to unwanted chemicals. (9)

Recent studies have shown than most oat products contain a small amount of glyphosate. There is a class action lawsuit against General Mills regarding the content of glyphosate in the cereal Cheerios. (10)

Glyphosate is so ubiquitous that it is now showing up even in organic foods, in the air and in the rain. But the more it is used, more weeds that it is intended to kill become immune to it. What do the users do - they use even more (about three pounds per American per year).

Food

The cancer research arm of the World Health Organization has found that "based on research on human exposure in the U.S., Canada and Sweden and on animal studies that found what the agency called 'convincing evidence' that the chemical caused cancer in laboratory animals, and is probably carcinogenic to humans." (11) A recent lawsuit in California granted a man $289 million in damages for cancer caused by the use of RoundUp in his work as a school groundskeeper. Many more lawsuits are in the court system. (12) (13)

Who is Orange?

Another possible toxin is 2,4-D (Dicholorphenoxyacetic acid), a component of Agent Orange. Agent Orange was widely used in Vietnam. Veterans of that war are now suffering cancers and heart disease that may be the result of that chemical. Lawsuits are currently pending. (14)

You may wisely ask why that toxin is currently be used extensively for weed control on our farms. According to data from the USDA (United States Department of Agriculture) projected use of this chemical is rising. (15)

One would think that the U.S. learned something from this disaster. But some companies continue to produce this chemical known as 2,4-D. It is increasing and is in our food. It is used on pasture and range land where our beef cattle craze. (Does your steak taste quite as good now?)

The fungus among us

Another increasing problem is the use of fungicides on our crops. This has led to a highly resistant fungus called *candida auris*. According to Tom Chiller who specializes in fungus infections and is head of the Fungal Branch for the Center for Disease Control and Prevention, it is becoming a global issue. Currently it strikes mostly people in nursing homes, hospitals and those with a weakened immune system. Drug resistant cases have shown up in the U.S. in New York, New Jersey, Illinois and Florida. Especially virulent, it kills 50 per cent of those infected within 90 days. (16)

Believed to have started in Asia, it has spread *"like wildfire"* according to Dr. Shawn Lockhart, a fungal disease expert at the Centers for Disease Control and Prevention. It requires extreme cleaning methods to get rid of it in hospital rooms. This seems like yet another reason to go organic.

In 2020, the coronavirus pandemic has taught us how difficult it is to prevent infection.

To *"bee"* or not to bee

If the bee disappeared off the face of the earth, man would only have four years left to live.

— *Maurice Maeterlinck, The Life of the Bee*

The lowly bee is not only known for its primary product, honey, and for its nasty sting. Bees and other insects are essential for pollinating crops. In fact, bees are responsible for at least one-third of the food that we eat. (17)

Unfortunately, bees are being killed off by the billions. The reason is the heavy use of pesticides in the farming industry.

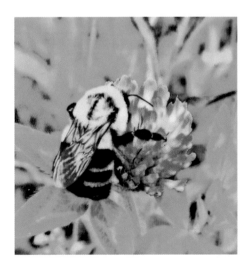

Lawns are another problem. They are responsible for a vast amount of acreage in the U.S. More pesticides we use on these, more insects that are essential to life will "bite the dust."

Food

It's a bug's life, or not

Not only bees but many other insects are becoming extinct. According to new research by scientists Francisco Sanchez-Bayoa and Kris A. G. Wyckhuys, "more than 40% of insect species are declining and a third are endangered...the mass of insects is falling by a precipitous 2.5% a year." (18)

According to Theunis Bates, Managing Editor, *The Week*, "a new study had found that insect biomass - the weight of all bugs on Earth combined- is dropping by a staggering 2.5 percent a year, largely because of pesticide use, habitat destruction, and climate change." (19)

Why does this matter? Troublesome as they are when we are outdoors, insects are essential to human life. Many birds are dependent on insects for food. Pollinating insects are obviously important in growing fruits and vegetables. Also, some insects are important because they eat pests that destroy crops.

The ladybug is one example. According to *National Geographic* for kids: "Most people like [ladybugs] because they are pretty, graceful, and harmless to humans. But farmers love them because they eat aphids and other plant-eating pests." (20)

Prof. John Losey, associate professor of entomology at Cornell University, founded the Lost Ladybug Project in 2000. It began in cooperation with 4-H Cooperative Extension Master Gardeners. Interest expanded and students in elementary schools in New York State started searching for rare ladybugs. The number of spots is important. As a result, an interesting school project extended to other states and funding from the National Science Foundation made more expansion possible.

A grassroots effort has grown to the point that anyone in North America can take part. See DiscoverLife.org or your local 4-H to learn more. If you see a ladybug, take a photograph, not a fly swatter. (21)

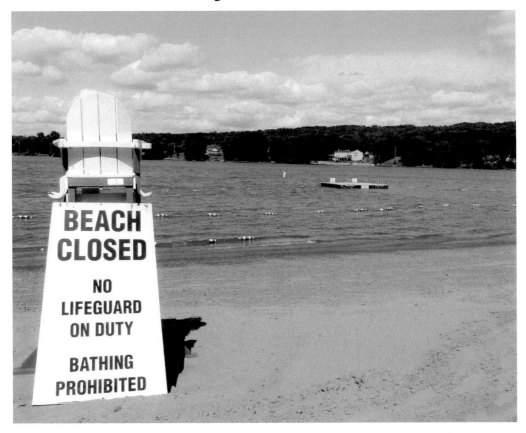

This beach near Syracuse, New York was closed for a time in summer 2019.

Get slimed

Lakes are being threatened by the Red Tide. This threat is cause by a fast-growing type of algae that loves phosphorus. Phosphorus comes from the runoff of fertilizers used primarily on farmland, golf courses and lawns as well as runoff of manure from nearby farms. (22) Residents of Toledo at the western end of Lake Erie were temporarily forced to stop using their water supply for a number of months in the summer. The green algae had made a huge glob of gelatinous material clogging the input of the water system supplying Toledo. (23)

The western side of Florida also had a major problem as algae in the Gulf of Mexico which shut down popular beaches during tourist season. Oneida Lake is a fairly large lake in central New York and it was shut down during the height of the summer season by the so-called Red Tide. Central New Yorkers treasure their short summer season so this had a major impact on swimming and fishing in the lake.

Red Tide can be harmful to humans and dogs. If you accidentally ingest seafood that has been infected by the algae that causes Red Tide can cause nausea, vomiting and diarrhea, as well as respiratory problems. It can cause neurological symptoms, especailly in dogs.(24)

In 2020, many beaches have been closed due to concerns about coronavirus spread.

Politics enters the door

The huge chemical manufacturers have a large stake in keeping things as they are with the many chemicals used increasingly in farming and on lawns. The equipment manufacturers want to sell large and expensive equipment to food producers. The food companies want food that is easily produced and garners huge profits for them. All of these groups have the money to pay for lobbyists to influence state government officials and the members of U.S. Congress. They have money to advertise and influence public opinion.

We are voters who can influence the way food is produced through voting and by the food we choose.

Hint:

Avoid chemicals if possible

Sally West Carman

Food

Part Two
Food Production

Food

Chapter three
A little dirt is good for you

It is our collective and individual responsibility to preserve and tend to the environment in which we all live.
          — Dalai Lama

Despite all your mother told you about keeping clean, the soil surrounding us is vitally important to our well-being. Healthy soil builds healthy crops and nourishes the people of the world.

Plants have the capacity to pull carbon into the soil out of the air. By increasing the amount of carbon in the soil, the percentage of carbon dioxide in the atmosphere can be reduced. According to Josh Tickell in *Kiss the Ground,* the world's soils contain 1,500 gigatons of carbon as a fixed stockpile. (1) Thus, if we can increase the carbon in the soil each year by even a small percent, we will be improving the soil and fighting climate change at the same time.

Sustainable farms are possible

Part of the philosophy of moving forward is by moving back. This means returning to some of the farming methods of the past. Currently more and more of the land in the United States is owned by corporations and very large family farms. Small family farms are finding it increasingly difficult to pay the bills with ever-decreasing profits.

The interests of the large agri-businesses are squeezing out the small farmers. Cargill is one of the largest privately-owned companies in the United States, and helped promote the use of high-fructose corn syrup, as well as owning many agricultural and non-agricultural companies. Large companies have so much influence that they can impact the manner in which farm bills are written. (2)

The federal governmental programs devised to supplement the income of farmers in lean years are being sucked up by these giant producers to increase their already hefty profits. (3)

No-till puts gold in the till

Perhaps we can convince our farmers that a new revolution in farming methods can be profitable. One method that seems revolutionary now, but was the original way of farming, is to eliminate plowing of the fields. Plowing allows the good topsoil to blow away, thereby putting carbon dioxide (that climate change agent) into the air. This is taking the precious carbon stored in the earth, essential for growing food, and making a greenhouse gas out it, thus warming the earth.

Also, plowing destroys the important ecosystem that we can't see beneath the surface. It also makes the soil less able to hold water and gases, thus causing runoff and compact soil. The compact soil cannot absorb all the water used to irrigate. (4)

The fungus among us

There are more microorganisms and crawly things beneath the surface than people above the surface. They are not attractive, but they are essential to breaking down the nutrients essential to the growth of the food we need to survive. Instead we use heavy and expensive machines and pricey artificial chemicals to supply what nature provides for free.

Microorganisms are becoming increasingly prominent as more research is done on their importance in agriculture. There are machines that have been developed to save some of these tiny but mighty creatures. This equipment can combine the old method of

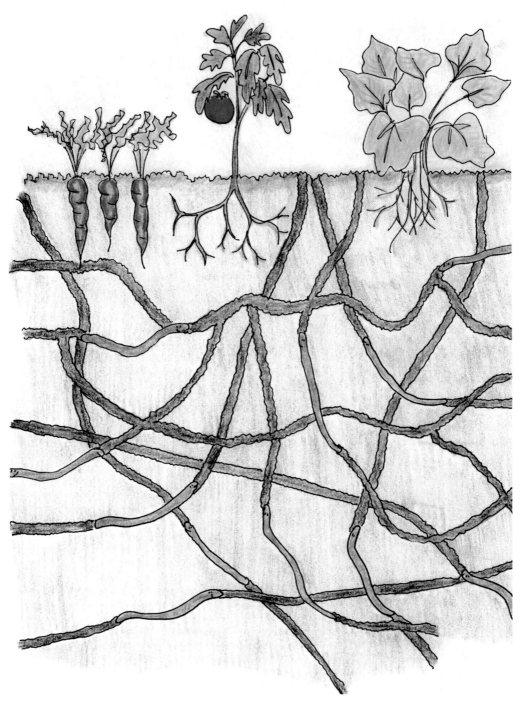

There are millions of microorganisms beneath the topsoil which are essential to the growth of our food. They are ugly but essential. Illustration by Susan Reardon

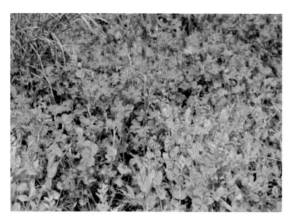

Cover crops nourish the soil by adding nitrogen and other nutrients.

tilling with sustainable farming methods. Rototilling can be done in strips so that paths between are undisturbed. (5)

Permaculture takes advantage of sustainable methods that have been shown to work. One of these is the use of raised beds. Using layers of mulch, compost and topsoil, a long furrow is planted with the desired crop. It also helps with drainage in rain-prone climates. The farm where I obtain my produce uses this method. (6)

Last fall I toured an urban garden project in Utica, New York where teenagers were being trained in these techniques.

Unfortunately, many of these methods are labor-intensive. Creative farmers have developed some ingenious techniques. Some machines poke holes in the ground in order to plant individual bulbs such as for garlic and potatoes, or for transplanting from seedlings grown in greenhouses.

Look for the four-leaf clover

Cover crops are another essential, but often forgotten method of enriching our soil for more growth of crops. Various types of clover and other plants have long been known to nourish the soil by pulling nitrogen from the air and incorporating it in the land. Many different cover crops are used depending on the growing zone. Heartier ones such as hairy vetch (doesn't sound very pretty does it?) are necessary in the northern regions. These also attract beneficial insects and control erosion. (7)

Andy Linder, a farmer in Minnesota, was able to retrofit a spraying machine to serve as a seeder of cover crops. He found that there was "less soil erosion, less compaction, increased water drainage, better soil structure, and increased weed suppression") by using this natural method of nourishing the soil. (8)

By rotating productive crops with cover crops the integrity of the soil can be maintained. This provides a natural method of fertilization that doesn't require artificial chemicals.

Don't put all your "eggs" in one basket

This philosophy works in food production much as it works in investing money. Planting a variety of crops provides some insurance against a bad year for one of them. Sometimes the others can take up the slack. This is ideal for the small farmer and one way to win against the huge, one-crop industrial operations. Local operations that provide farmers' markets and

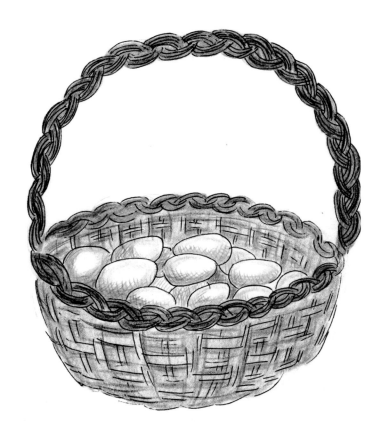

A variety of crops can supplement each other. Even adding some dairy cows can add natural manure, and trees can provide water retention. Illustration by Susan Reardon

farmers using sustainable methods generally follow this principle. (More in chapter nine.)

Also, combining different crops that like each other can be a blessing. Crops such as buckwheat, peas, and sweet potatoes are some examples. Some farmers have learned that adding dairy cows can produce manure for natural fertilizer. (9)

The farm-to-table movement is a somewhat new and growing concept. A well-known example is Blue Hill, in New York City. The chef, Dan Barber, owns this very popular restaurant. The cuisine utilizes produce and livestock from Stone Barns Center for Food and Agriculture, twenty miles north of the city on land donated by David Rockefeller. Barber expanded to another restaurant, Blue Hill at Stone Barns. (10)

He attributes his success to the succulence of the produce produced by sustainable methods. These methods rely on natural techniques rather than artificial fertilizers and soil-depleting strategies.

Dandelions are flowers

Fertilizers, as discussed in the last chapter, have become ubiquitous. Home owners are just as much to blame as the gigantic producers. We are so brainwashed to expect our lawns to look perfect that we shovel on the chemical fertilizers. When it rains, these chemicals leach into our streams and onto our neighbor's properties. If we can change our values to accept some diversity in our surroundings, we can help our earth in at least a small way. Appreciate the beautiful yellow dandelion flowers and pick the greens for salad as our grandmothers once did (assuming no pesticides or animals have been there first).

Milkweed need not be pasteurized

Fields of wild flowers should be encouraged. They provide

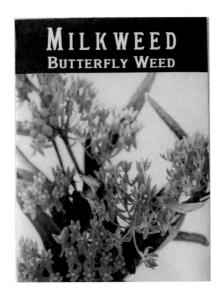

a natural way to feed important pollinators as mentioned in Chapter two. Milkweed, even a small line of plants around the field or garden, provides the essential food for the beautiful Monarch Butterfly. These butterflies are quickly headed for extinction if we do not do something to prevent it. (11)

Variety is the spice of life

The bottom line is diversity seems to be the key to better soil, more profitability and saving some important species upon which we depend.

Hint

Encourage sustainable farming by buying sustainably grown and organic products.

Food

Chapter four
Corny is no joke

The earth will not continue to offer its harvest, except with faithful stewardship. We cannot say we love the land and then take steps to destroy it for use by future generations.
                                                    — Pope John Paul II

Politics and farms don't mix

Unfortunately, federal legislation has a large effect on the crops that are grown. The use of subsidies for farmers was a good idea with unintended consequences. These subsidies single out certain crops to be encouraged while others are ignored.

The rich get richer

According to Chris Edwards in his paper on *Agricultural Subsidies*, "about 39 percent of the nation's 2.1 million farms receive subsidies, with the lion's share of the handouts going to the largest producers of corn, soybeans, wheat, cotton and rice." (1)

There is a farm lobby with enough clout to keep these subsidies in business. The problem is that the majority of handouts go to corn, soybeans and wheat, not to fruit and vegetable growers. There are no income limits on the recipients of these subsidies, so millionaires and billionaires can reap the profits. They do not lower food prices or benefit the small, family farmers.

Subsidize me

Government subsidies to farmers also have a large impact on what gets grown and who grows it. The public has little knowledge of the way in which their tax dollars are spent on subsidies.

The idea of subsidies is to help farmers even out their income in a highly fluctuating market. This means that money is given to match a set price for a commodity, such as a bushel of corn, and if it doesn't sell for that, the difference will be made up by the federal government. It was devised as a way to keep farmers from going bankrupt.

Where have all the farmers gone

Sadly, most of the subsidies go to very large farms. According to Adam Andrzejewski, a contributor to Forbes on-line and founder of OpenTheBooks.com, "since 2008, the top 10 farm subsidy recipients each received an average of $18.2 million." (2)

Tina Haspel writing in the *Washington Post* in March 2018 stated "in many cases about half the money went to farmers with household incomes over $150,000... three times the median household income at the time." (3) At the same time, farmers all around us are going bankrupt.

One result is that large industrial farms focus on large field crops, and not fruits and vegetables that naturally have more nutrients. The favored crops discourage crop rotation and increased use of fertilizers.

Also, another unintended consequence of subsidies is that it favors certain crops and larger farm operations. Corn has been one of the highly-subsidized crops. The use of ethanol in gasoline is one reason. Corn is a source of ethanol, an alternative to oil. That sounds good. However, cars still need a mixture of oil and ethanol unless they are totally redesigned. Electric cars are becoming more common and will change the importance of ethanol.

Corn is also a source of high-fructose corn syrup. It has become ubiquitous in so many foods. If consumers don't read ingredient labels carefully, they will the miss the fact that high-fructose corn syrup is just another form of sugar. Unfortunately, the only positive effect sugar has in our diet is energy. It has no vitamins, minerals or micro-nutrients. Since all food supplies us with energy, albeit more slowly, sugar is only an easy way to add to the waistline. (Read your labels.)

And most of the profits go to the distributors. For example, the dairy farmer reaps only a small percentage of the cost of the gallon of milk we buy at the store. According to an article in *Agweek* in July 2018, "a few years ago, U.S. farmers were making about $18 for every 100 pounds of milk they produced, which equates to about 11.6 gallons. Now, they're getting around $15."(4) Each year the amount that farmers receive is less and less. In extreme cases, farmers have had to pour precious milk down the drain.

Studies have shown the value of organic milk. However, the cost of being certified organic is as much as $3000 per year to the farmer. Even if he or she insists on organic practices, this is often not cost-effective for the "little guy," the individual farmer. Plus, the farmer must find a place that will process the organic milk. One local farmer I spoke to said that the business that processes her milk has to completely clean the equipment before processing the organic milk to prevent contamination.

The cost of equipment needed to support most current farming practices is astronomical, putting the farmer deeply in debt and cutting deeply into profits. Organic farming that requires less equipment may be more profitable in the long run, but is usually highly labor-intensive.

Corporate farms "eat" small farms

As running a farm profitably becomes more and more difficult, farmers are forced to give up. They have to sell their land and equipment. Many sons and daughters don't want to stay on the farm to help out because it is demanding work for a small reward. Many others love the independence of farming, the idea of being one's own boss and producing something of value.

The changing weather and climate change make for variable growing conditions. The smaller farm is not able to "weather" these changes during the lean years. Droughts in the Midwest and West in recent years have been devastating, and are likely to get worse. Huge irrigation systems enable the large farms to survive. However, this leads to major water shortages.

Hot weather dries out the soil, especially with indiscriminate plowing. Plowing spews more carbon dioxide into the atmosphere, as mentioned above.

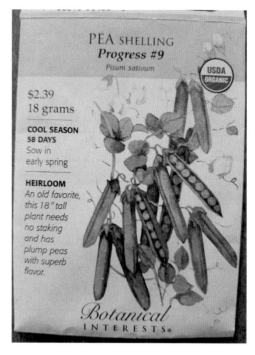

Organic seeds are difficult to find. These came from a farm store in Colorado.

GMO = get money out of the ground

Genetically modified (GMO) crops have gotten a lot of press. Are they a good or bad thing? We don't know yet what the long-term effects of these will be. We have to ask, why were they developed?

They were developed to withstand the use of herbicides and pesticides on the crops. (One of my friends was one of the early developers and she had all good intentions of helping to feed the world.) The idea was to rid the fields of invasive weeds and crop-eating pests. It became easier to have a larger yield with less person-power needed.

The problem is the unintended consequences. Those pesky weeds and pests developed resistance to the chemicals being used. This required the use of more chemicals at more expense and more danger, both to those who spread the chemicals and to those who consume the crops.

These special GMO seeds also tend to spread to land where they are not wanted. In addition, the big corporations decided to control the seeds, so that it becomes increasingly difficult to obtain seeds that are not GMO. Fewer producers are left that sell so-called "heritage" seeds.

And what about taste tests? These seeds have not been developed for taste. They have been developed for profit. We start to forget what a vegetable grown "naturally" tastes like. That large garden my dad lovingly maintained across the street from our upscale, suburban home near Chicago taught me to love vegetables because they tasted wonderful straight from the garden. My dad always said "Boil the water before you pick the corn."

Farmers markets in season can still make this possible - more about the later.

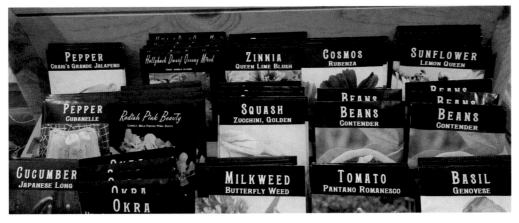

This rack holds a variety of organic seeds and was found at a gift shop.

Food

How we vote, not only at the ballot box but with our wallets, can make a difference. Our food choices influence what is produced.

Hint

Buy organic milk, grain, fruits and vegetables.
Shop at famer's markets

Chapter five
What's the beef?

The hardest part of returning to a truly healthy environment may be changing the current totally unsustainable heavy-meat-eating culture of increasing numbers of people around the world. But we must try. We must make a start, one by one.
    — Jane Goodall, Harvest for Hope: A Guide to Mindful Eating

Cows are vegetarians

Cows are born with the natural ability to eat things humans cannot. That is because they are lucky to have four stomachs.

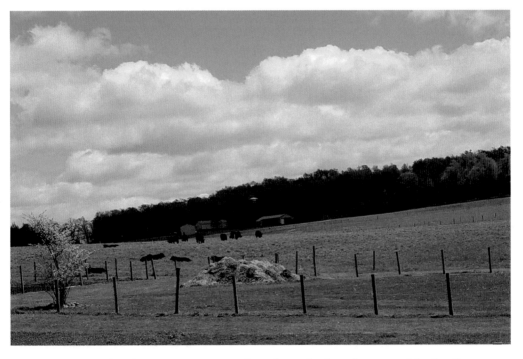

These cows prefer the green grass rather than the hay just outside the fence.

This enables them to chew on grass and turn it into milk for dairy cows and steaks for beef cattle.

Cows can be very picky. They love nice, green grass, but refuse to eat certain nasty weeds. They can survive on hay, but it is not their favorite.

Farmers who are concerned about the environment and growing healthy food, maintain large pastures of green grass. They move their cows to new grasslands when one field gets chewed to the roots and needs to recover. Some farmers have found that portable electric fences are a good way to steer their steers into greener pastures. They don't keep their cows confined to a stable.

Cows need mouthwash

Unfortunately, cows breathe out a form of methane. Methane is a potent greenhouse gas that is responsible for 25% of air pollution, and is much more potent than carbon dioxide. Some organic farmers have tried various methods to reduce this methane, with little success. Of course, methane caused by industry is also a great problem.

A manure lagoon is no sand beach

What goes in one end, comes out the other end. If you have ever followed a tractor pulling a manure spreader, you know what an odoriferous load it is. Manure from cows can be a good natural fertilizer as long as certain standards are maintained. Unfortunately, in some large industrial operations, this byproduct is dumped into a large, pond-like depression. This is not an area for swimming. It is a fertile ground for all sorts of insect pests.

Livestock contributes to the pollution of our global water supply and is "responsible for 37 percent of pesticide use, 55 percent of erosion, and 50 percent of the volume of antibiotics consumed." (1)

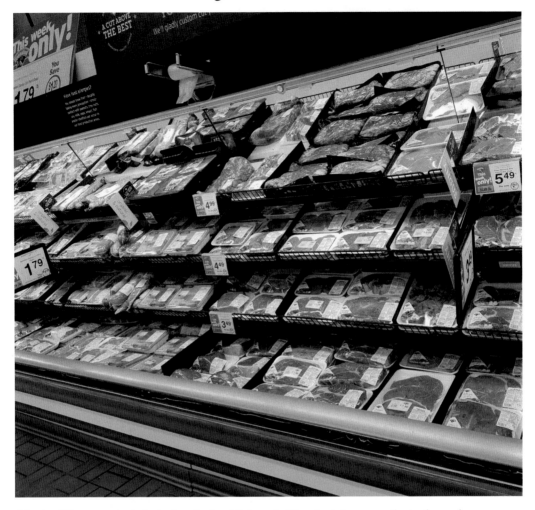

Most of the meat aisle is loaded with beef. The butchers and stockyards are kept hidden. It takes effort to find the non-red meat options.

Do cows have emotions?

For a time, **mad-cow** disease was a major worry as cattle had to be put to death to prevent the spread of mad-cow disease. It results from improper methods used in beef cattle operations. Many cows were put to death in Great Britain to limit the problem, though recently this has not been considered a major issue. (2)

Food

Watch what you say

The political connection cannot be ignored. Even the great Oprah Winfrey got in trouble for emphasizing some of the problems of red meat on her show. She had to back down when she urged people to stop eating hamburgers on her show in April 16, 1996. She was taken to court by the National Cattleman's Beef Association. **Money has a loud voice.** Even though she won the case, Oprah no longer has much to say about beef. (3)

Eat meat at your own risk

Despite what the advertising says, red meat includes: beef, lamb, goat, pork, venison, dark-meat poultry and poultry skin. These all contain more "artery-clogging saturated fat than does skinless, white-meat poultry and fish." (4)

In addition to the environmental risk, red meat has a substantial health risk. Those meats that are processed, including bacon, luncheon meat, salami, hot dogs and sausage, have additional risks. A longitudinal study conducted over four years by Dr. Frank Hu of the Harvard School of Public Health showed an increased number of deaths from cancer and heart disease. The study found that *"one additional serving per day of unprocessed red meat over the course of the study raised the risk of total mortality by 13%. An extra serving of processed red meat (such as bacon, hot dogs, sausage and salami) raised the risk by 20%.... Substituting fish, poultry, nuts, legumes, low-fat dairy and whole grains—for red meat could lower the risk of mortality by 7% to 19%."* (5)

A diet composed in large part of red meat is also *linked to many health problems such as heart disease, type 2 diabetes and colorectal cancer.* (6)

A study done in the United Kingdom reported by the National Health Service found that red meat increases the incidence of bowel cancer. (7) This is based on a study by The Scientific Advisory Committee on Nutrition that focused on the consumption of red and processed meat. Their recommendation is to eat no more than 70 grams a day. A slice of ham has 23 grams and a quarter pound-beef burger has 78 grams. (8)

According to a recent study in the *Journal of the American Medical Association,* red meat produces a substance when it is digested in the body which puts people who eat it at a higher risk of "both cardiovascular disease and early death." (9) (10) The product of metabolism is known by the acronym TMAO (tri-methylamine–oxide). High levels of this have been linked to chronic kidney disease and heart failure.

That super-sized burger doesn't sound quite so appetizing now, does it.

Save the rainforest.

Unfortunately, not only health concerns are the issue. **Beef is one of the major contributors to climate change.** The recent fires and major destruction of the Amazon Rainforest has been caused by ranchers in Brazil. In order to open more land for grazing beef cattle (as well as for soybeans), they start fires which spread rapidly. U.S. citizens are major consumers of this beef.

In order to produce a half pound of hamburger, it takes 55 square miles of rainforest. It also requires 1200 gal. of water. (11) (More about water scarcity in chapter seven.)

The rainforests of South America are a long way from us so why do we care?   The Amazon rainforest provides as much as 20% of the oxygen in the atmosphere of the entire globe. It is also home to millions of species, many endangered. The tops of these ancient trees support an entire ecosystem - still largely unexplored. These trees have traditionally been a great sink for carbon dioxide, pulling it out of the atmosphere and returning much needed oxygen. Once gone, these ancient trees cannot be replaced. (More about trees in chapter eight.)

However, the beef industry has a huge amount of influence. The vested interest of large producers is to convince us that red meat is good for us. Though it is a source of protein, it is also a major source of saturated fat, the bad stuff. Not only that, it is expensive to buy.

When you choose what to eat, you are voting in the consumer marketplace.

Hint

Cut down on, or eliminate, red meat in your diet.

Chapter six
Something is fishy

When the last tree has been cut down, the last fish caught, the last river poisoned, only then will we realize that one cannot eat money.
— Native American Saying

To tell you the truth, I have been putting off working on this chapter. Fish is not my favorite dish, though I usually eat it at least once a week. When I was growing up in the Midwest, we did not always have a freezer, and fish was not as available as it is now. However, many parts of the world survive on fish, and over-fishing is becoming a serious problem.

Ocean hot tub

The rising temperatures are causing the oceans, as well as the air, to warm. These temperature changes affect the fish as they are very sensitive to the water temperature. This means fish migrate to cooler waters farther north. Salmon are particularly affected as they require a certain temperature range in which to spawn.

Much of the salmon that we eat in the U.S. comes from Alaska. The normal habitat of the salmon is being disrupted by dams, dikes and pipelines. Also, the pollution caused by industrial plants is an issue. We have polluted the waterways with sewage and other waste, including plastic. (More about that later.)

Salmon also require plankton and krill to eat. Krill makes a compound called astaxanthin which is essential to their growth and gives them their reddish hue. Humans gain this antioxidant that fights inflammation when they eat salmon. These fish also have high levels of omega-3s (see below).

The mercury is rising

Not only is the temperature rising because of climate change, but the mercury level is also rising in the fish population. According to an article in *Scientific American*, "...human industrial activity (such as coal-fired electricity generation, smelting and the incineration of waste) ratchets up the amount of airborne mercury which eventually finds its way into lakes, rivers and the ocean, where it is gobbled up by unsuspecting fish and other marine life." (1)

The problem is much greater in larger fish who dine on smaller fish. This concentrates the amount of mercury in the larger fish. According to the newsletter *Healthline*, high levels of mercury can cause significant health problems. These may include brain

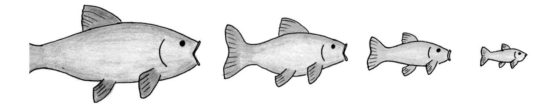

Small fish are eaten by larger fish, which are eaten by ever larger fish, thus concentrating the mercury. Illustratoion by Susan Reardon.

problems and diseases such as Alzheimer's, Parkinsonism, Autism and even depression. (2)

Fish to avoid, especially if you are pregnant or planning to become pregnant, include swordfish, tuna steaks and King mackerel. The fish lowest in mercury include shrimp, scallops, oysters and salmon. Fish in the moderate range are haddock, cod and whiting. (3) (4)

However, eating fish can be an important part of a healthy diet because fish contains omega-3 fatty acids.

What is the deal about the Omegas?

Omega-3 is good for you, you have heard it. It is a vital fatty acid, which means your body must consume it and can't make it on its own. Fish is the best source. Of the types mentioned above, salmon has the highest concentration of omega-3s. According to Paul Greenberg in *American Catch, a one-ounce portion of cooked salmon contains eight hundred milligrams of omega-3s.* Salmon is also high in magnesium, potassium, selenium and B vitamins, so it is a real bargain. (5)

Omega-6 is important too. The balance of omega-3 and omega-6 is vital. Keep in mind that your omega-6 to omega-3 ratio can cause problems, as a diet low in omega-3s but high in omega-6s can increase inflammation and your risk of disease. Vegetable oils are one of the main sources of omega-6. Poultry, eggs and nuts are other sources.

Fish oil pills are being touted in the media. However, not all omega-3s are equal. There are three types: ALA, DHA and EPA. ALA and linoleic acid must be obtained from the diet. ALA is found in flaxseed, soybean and canola oils. DHA and EPA are produced poorly by the liver and thus also are best consumed in food. (6)

Taking a fish oil pill may not be the answer. They vary greatly in quality, and in composition. If you don't eat any fish, a prescription fish oil pill is probably the best.

However, there are other sources for those folks who hate fish. Flax seeds are one alternative and are also very high in fiber, vitamin E, magnesium and other nutrients. They have a great omega-6 to omega-3 ratio compared to most oily plant seeds. Chia seeds are another option. Walnuts are also great sources of omega 3s and are a source of copper, manganese, and vitamin E.

Surprise, Brussel sprouts are another source of those important omega-3s. (7) (8)

Go get those omegas!

Where have all the fish gone?

Unfortunately, over-fishing has caused a sharp decline in the fish population. The number of fish farms has risen in response to the high demand. However, the water in these farms can become easily polluted with fish excrement if not maintained properly. If you have an aquarium, you are aware of the problem and the need for frequent cleaning.

The U.S. is surrounded by oceans and streams meander through the land. But we have moved away from fish as part of our diet, consuming burgers instead of fish sandwiches. Fish do not require fertilizer to grow, or vast grasslands to graze, or pesticides to kill bugs. Therefore, they are friendly to our environment.

There is a rising interest in fish as part of our diets. Hopefully this will continue.

Hint

Eat more fish, flax seeds and chia seeds.

Chapter seven
Water, water everywhere, but not a drop to drink

Because, underneath all of this is the real truth we have been avoiding: climate change isn't an "issue" to add to the list of things to worry about, next to health care and taxes. It is a civilizational wake-up call. A powerful message—spoken in the language of fires, floods, droughts, and extinctions—telling us that we need an entirely new economic model and a new way of sharing this planet. Telling us that we need to evolve.
— Naomi Klein

Most of the earth is covered by oceans. Why is drinking water something we often buy in a bottle instead of pouring from the tap? Some parts of the United States are suffering severe drought, while other parts are drowning in severe flooding.

Build your shore house on stilts

This has even become a national security threat. The Naval Base at Norfolk, VA is sinking into the ocean and the U.S. Navy is working on solutions. According to *James Balogh* in his documentary, *The Human Element,* "this is the largest base in the country and it is disappearing before our eyes." Balogh is a photo-journalist who has been traveling the world to visually document the changing conditions. (1)

This Base, the oldest in the U.S. (built in 1799) had to be closed nine times in ten years because of the rising ocean. (2) It is only one of 128 military bases that are threatened with rising seas. (3)

Food

Because the glaciers are melting, the water going into the ocean is increasing at an alarming rate, causing ocean levels to rise. All the communities along the coasts are the most endangered. Florida is in continual danger because it is surrounded by water on both sides. This popular retirement state floats on caves of water underneath. As the water is being drawn from the ground to meet the needs of the ever-increasing population, sinkholes are opening up unexpectedly. According to *Smithsonian Magazine.* "they occur more frequently in Florida than any other state."(4)

Southern Manhattan and Staten Island in New York City, the largest city in the U.S., are also in grave danger of being inundated. The city is actually constructing barriers in its underground subway system to try to hold back the tide of water expected with the next hurricane. (5) Some people in New York, New Jersey, Florida and especially in Puerto Rico, are still recovering from the last hurricanes that blew through.

Send fracking packing

The ever-increasing need for oil and gas has caused companies to build costly extraction sites to release the oil far underground. In order to do this requires millions and billions of gallons of precious water which has been laced with dangerous chemicals. The water is forced underground under tremendous pressure to release the fossil fuel buried in the ground. This poisoned water cannot economically be recovered and fills huge, recovery ponds of sludge.

According to LiveScience.com, "air pollution, groundwater contamination, health problems and surface water pollution are some of the negative effects of fracking." (6) Also, Parts of Oklahoma where fracking has become a major industry have been threatened with a new raft of earthquakes. (7) We are proving again that you *should not mess with Mother Nature.*

The poison in us

The infrastructure of many of towns and cities is built upon a mass of old lead-containing pipes. Some of this lead can leach into our drinking water. Other chemicals from fertilizers are washed from farmland into our streams and lakes. Water main breaks cause "boil water" directives in many towns. (8)

We try to fight this by buying water in plastic bottles. If you read the label, much of this has come from municipal water systems. Some company takes everything out of the water and then has to add something to give it taste, and perhaps some minerals to make it sell.

Unfortunately some elements such as Bisphenol A (BPA) in the plastic can leach into the water. Leaving your plastic bottle in a hot car is especially dangerous. (9)

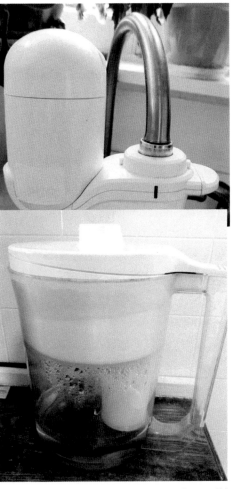

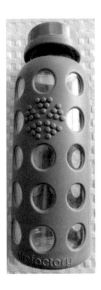

Use water bottles and filters, not bottled water.

Think about how all that plastic is manufactured - from oil. Think about the millions of plastic bottles bobbing in the ocean and using space in landfills. They don't break down over centuries. Do we really need water that comes from the Island of Fiji?

My solution is to buy a filter for the faucet at my sink, and a water container with a filter for the refrigerator and the upstairs bathroom. It saves a lot of money, and time lugging water bottles.

Chemicals everywhere

Another concern found not only in municipal drinking water but also in private wells is PFASs. This stands for: per- and poly-fluoroalkyl substances (PFAS) ...a group of man-made chemicals that have been in use since the 1940s. (9) They have been found in cookware, food packaging and are part of the firefighting foam used at airports. The best treatment is activated charcoal, and there are federal funds available to deal with this problem. It is a good idea to have your own water supply tested for contaminants.

See more about drinking water in Chapter ten.

Hints

Oppose fracking in your state
Use water filters
Get your drinking water tested

Chapter eight
A tree grows in your backyard

They paved paradise
And put up a parking lot

> -Joni Mitchell in *Big Yellow Taxi*, 1970

Trees are a triple treat

Trees provide a source of food. They provide the apples, pears, oranges and other fruits that we love. They also provide various types of nuts: almonds, chestnuts, walnuts and my favorite pecans. Maple trees give us maple syrup through boiling of their sap.

Trees provide shade in the hotter months. They also enable shade-loving plants to grow. They hold water in the soil preventing flooding.

However, we don't usually think of trees as saving our planet. Trees have a tremendous capacity to take the CO_2 that we breathe and that factories exhale, and turn it into oxygen that is essential for lives. Trees can help fight the stampede toward ever-increasing climate change.

Johnny Appleseed was a hero

The story goes that Johnny Appleseed traveled the country spreading apple seeds where they would grow into trees. The real Johnny was John Chapman (1774 - 1845) and he actually planted nurseries surrounded by fences to protect them from livestock. These were spread throughout Pennsylvania, Indiana and Ohio. There is even a museum dedicated to him in Urbana, Ohio. (1)

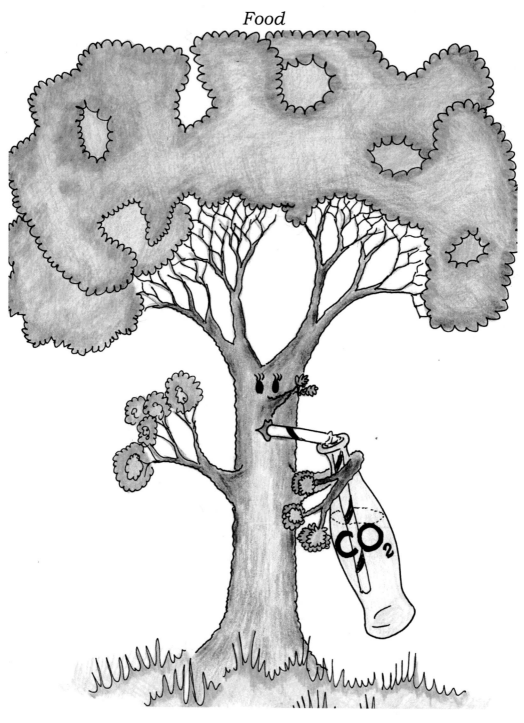

A tree has many benefits for the environment. It sucks up carbon dioxide (that greenhouse gas) and produces oxygen for life. Also, trees retain water to prevent flooding and provide shade. Illustration by Susan Reardon.

However, there is some question as to Johnny's saintliness. According to Michael Pollan in *The Botany of Desire: A Plant's Eye View of the World,* the apples planted by Johnny were not the edible type and could only be used for cider. That hard cider may have made him very popular in cabins throughout the east. (2)

An apple a day keeps the doctor away?

There is no doubt that apples are healthy, providing fiber and many important nutrients. The problem is that many producers use large quantities of poisonous sprays to kill pests. Recently I was talking to a local farmer who had to quit his job at a local orchard. The reason was that the constantly spraying of chemicals made his entire face swell up, forcing him to retire. Then he started his own CSA farm a mile from the orchard (more about that in a later chapter). The sad thing is that the high-spraying orchard sells fruit and vegetables at our local farmer's market all summer.

Wouldn't you prefer apples with some blemishes, rather than coated with chlorpyrifos, a highly toxic pesticide? According to Friends of the Earth, "It's part of a class of chemicals developed as a nerve gas by Nazi Germany. It has been linked to Parkinson's disease and lung cancer." (3)

Hawaii became the first state to ban chlorpyrifos in June 2018. "Governor David Ige signed Senate Bill 3095 into law, which now prohibits the use of restricted pesticides within 100 feet of a school during normal hours beginning January 1st. It also requires a permit to use pesticides containing the neurotoxin, chlorpyrifos, as an active ingredient and totally bans the chemical in 2023." (4)

One of the most widely used insecticides in the U.S. and around the world, chlorpyrifos has been identified in cases of asthma and various lung problems, especially among young people. According to a study at Columbia University, prenatal exposure is especially dangerous and *"may lead to irreversible changes in the brain of the child. (5)*

In summer 2020, the NRDC announced: "In a huge win for public health, Corteva...has announced it will stop producing chlorpyrifos."(6) NRDC is working toward a federal ban on that chemical.

The alternative is to buy organic apples or ones produced using sustainable farming methods. Cutting off a few blemishes is a small price to pay for good health.

This applies to many other fruits as well. Especially in the case of fruits and vegetables where we eat the skin, such as strawberries, spinach, kale, pears, peaches and grapes. It is nearly impossible to wash off all of the chemicals. Look for organic fruit instead. (7)

Roasting chestnuts

Chestnuts are also one of the "fruits" of a tree. They are often found during the Christmas season, and are featured in Christmas. They are very tasty, but not so easy to roast. The secret is to put a tiny hole in each before putting them in the oven. I had a spectacular disaster one year with exploding chestnuts in my oven. Recently I found some in a package at my local natural food store where all the hard work had been done and they were ready to eat.

They take down trees and put up parking lots

Unfortunately, in many parts of the world trees are disappearing faster than new ones can grow. The lush Amazon River once lined by trees is becoming barren. As mentioned in Chapter five, the trees are quickly being chopped down and turned into firewood and farmland. The soybean crops and beef production are very profitable and a huge incentive causing this devastation. (8)

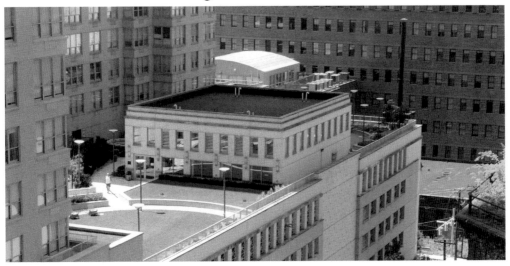

This view from my grandson's apartment in New Jersey shows a landscape atop a building.

In parts of Africa, trees are turned into charcoal and used for heat and cooking. There are efforts by several charitable organizations to supply stoves that do not require wood, and even some that use solar heat. (9)

Wildfires are another source of the decimation of trees, as well as houses. Dry conditions caused by climate change make trees susceptible to a tiny spark which can ignite an entire forest. The devastation in California is an example of the danger to life, livestock and homes. (10)

The aftermath of these wildfires has been giant mudslides when it rains, burying people, crops and houses. Planting trees and fast-growing ground cover seems the only solution.

Trees grow on skyscrapers

Each person can make a difference by planting one tree or more. The Arbor Foundation will even send you tree saplings for free. However, trees do require a significant amount of nurturing. You can find an arborist at a local college, or in New York, Cornell Cooperative Extension Agents will help.

Food

When I last visited New York City, I was surprised by the number of trees growing on the top of imposing skyscrapers. Amid all the concrete gloom, people needed to experience a bit of nature, and planted gardens on the rooftops. Also, an old railroad bed has been turned into a local tourist attraction, lined with plants and a place to walk above the traffic. Called the Highline, it has become very popular.

By being a little creative, perhaps you can add some extra bits of nature to your environment. Become a modern-day Johnny Appleseed. **Plant a tree!**

Hints

Support the Arbor Foundation
Plant a tree

Sally West Carman

Food

Part Three
Buying and storing food

Food

Chapter nine
Keep Mother Nature on your side

Odd as I am sure it will appear to some; I can think of no better form of personal involvement in the cure of the environment than that of gardening. A person who is growing a garden, if he is growing it organically, is improving a piece of the world. He is producing something to eat, which makes him somewhat independent of the grocery business, but he is also enlarging, for himself, the meaning of food and the pleasure of eating.
— Wendell Berry The Art of Compromise: the Agrarian Essays

Many ways to grow a radish

More and more people are finding the usefulness and enjoyment of small-scale gardens. This might be a small plot in the backyard, or a large container with one or two tomato plants. Even people living in apartments grow things on their balcony, or a shared space on the roof. They are learning to appreciate the vibrant taste of a vegetable fresh-picked, and the satisfaction of watching something grow and feeling responsible for its success.

More information about commercial greenhouses is outlined in Chapter fourteen

Water gardens in the kitchen

Known as hydroponics, growing small plants in a container lit by LED lights is possible on a countertop in your kitchen. Several companies make these, and will sell you pods complete with seeds, or plant-your-own pods which are made specifically for these gardens. These enclosed units have a small pump to

Food

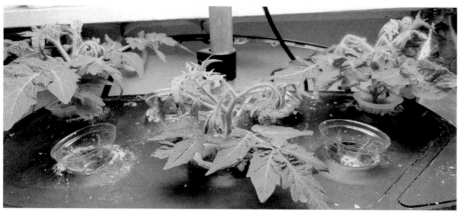

This shows the tomato plants starting to grow, with the results below.

aerate the water and do require a monthly dose of liquid plant food. They are especially good for growing herbs, lettuce, and cherry tomatoes. I had a tomato plant that lasted more than a year. I finally had to throw it out and start something new, even though it continued producing.

Some producers have actually started larger water-based gardens in greenhouses, growing items such as

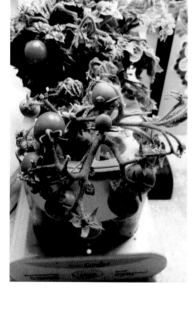

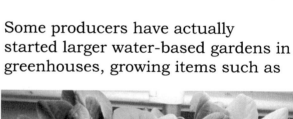

Lettuce is easily grown in a kitchen garden.

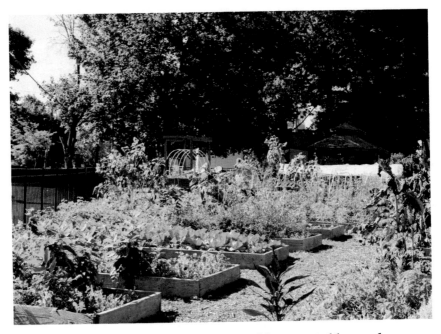

This community garden in the city provides vegetables and exercise for urban residents.

lettuce to sell to local restaurants. Even in Disney-world there is huge hydroponic greenhouse growing all types of plants. You can take a *behind the seeds* tour at their facility in Epcot in their *Living with the Land* building. It also includes fish farming. (1)

Community gardens

School groups are planting gardens on school grounds and teachers use this as a learning experience. One of these groups had a "pizza garden" planting the ingredients of a pizza and having a pizza party at the end of the summer.

Community groups are banding together to cultivate a plot in their neighborhood, sharing the tasks as well as the proceeds in the form of healthy vegetables. Friendships are formed as neighbors work together toward a common goal.

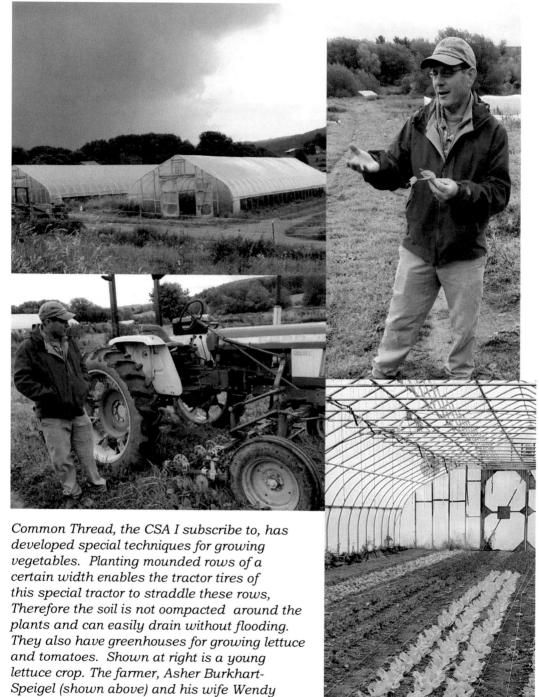

Common Thread, the CSA I subscribe to, has developed special techniques for growing vegetables. Planting mounded rows of a certain width enables the tractor tires of this special tractor to straddle these rows, Therefore the soil is not oompacted around the plants and can easily drain without flooding. They also have greenhouses for growing lettuce and tomatoes. Shown at right is a young lettuce crop. The farmer, Asher Burkhart-Speigel (shown above) and his wife Wendy take care of twenty acres in central New York with the help of a small staff. They also train young interns.

CSA - Community Supported Agriculture

This program known as CSA was developed in the 80s. Steven McFadden, who co-authored the first book on CSA, *Farms of Tomorrow*, estimated that there were at least 6000 CSAs in the U.S. in 2012, and the program is growing. The concept is to grow food on a cooperative basis without the use of herbicides, pesticides or artificial fertilizer. (2)

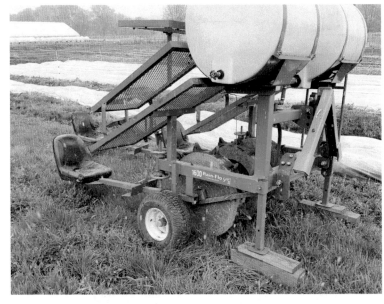

This resourceful CSA farmer put together this special planter for no-till farming.

The professional grower decides on the various crops to be grown each season, and sells shares in what will be produced. In some instances, the shareholders are responsible for helping during the growing season. In others, they merely need to pick up the produce once a week, either from the farm itself, or from a central pick-up location. (3)

The only downside is there is often no choice in what is produced. However, it will be fresh, in-season, and free of any poisons. Shareholders often share recipes for using the produce, and some even hold pot-luck dinners.

Food

The CSA I subscribe to does offer a choice of vegetables, and has shares of root crops during the winter. We attended their tour in the rain (guess

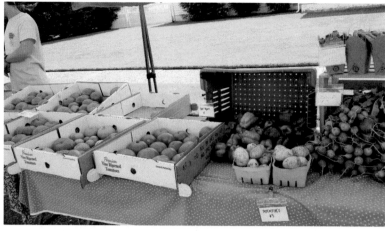

Farmlers markets in central New York and New Jersey

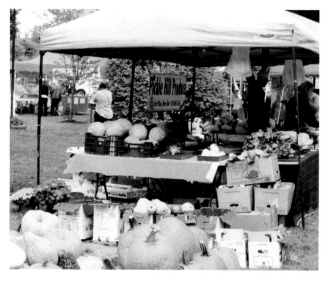

we were committed) and attended a pot-luck dinner.

Farmer's markets

Farmer's markets are becoming common in small and larger cities across the country. This enables farmers to sell directly to the public without a middle-man taking part of the profit. Consumers can buy fresher produce, and interact directly with the grower. Questions about farming practices will determine if artificial chemicals are used. In many cases vegetables are grown with sustainable farming methods because of the difficulty and expense of becoming certified as organic.

Farmer's markets are even taking place during the winter months in northern areas. Root crops that can be easily stored such as potatoes and beets are available in the winter. Maple syrup and crafts are other products.

Slow Food Movement

Perhaps a strange name for an environmental group, the Slow Food Movement encompasses many

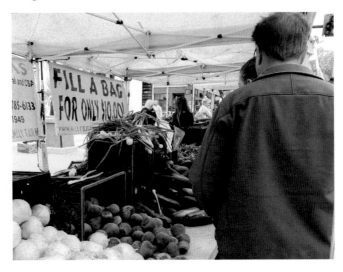

This is a farmer's market in Colorado.

aspects of environmental impacts of foods. I believe it means appreciating your food fully (eating slowly), understanding where it comes from and the impact that producing food has on our environment. A recent part of this is a move to legislate a "Green New Deal" by U.S. Congressional action.

Their goal (as elaborated on their website): "[is to begin] working collaboratively with farmers and ranchers in the United States to remove pollution and greenhouse gas emissions from the agricultural sector as much as is technologically feasible...by supporting family farming; by investing in sustainable farming and land-use practices that increase soil health; and by building a more sustainable food system that ensures universal access to healthy food... "(4)

They are proposing a Conservation Stewardship Program (CSP) which would reward farmers for activities that improve "soil, water, and air quality." A giant farm bill was passed in December 2018 which provides "funds for local farmers markets, research funds for organic farming, and money for organizations working to train the next generation of farmers." It also encourages cover crops. These seem like steps in the right direction. (5)

Food

Save the packaging and transportation cost

Finding ways of growing and buying directly are important for helping to solve environmental issues as well. The plastic wrap seen throughout the supermarket is avoided if you bring your own canvas bags. (We will address this in chapter eleven.)

The cost of transporting food, no matter how it is packaged, from distant parts of the U.S. and other countries is enormous. It also uses precious fossil fuels for trucks. Try to buy produce in-season and locally as much as possible. This avoids the transportation problem.

Hints

Buy in season
Shop at farmer's markets
Support a CSA

Chapter ten
Making food choices

'I have a strong feeling, that as a human being I owe the pot, and to the degree that one can give back to it one ought to.
  -Rev. Robert Fulghum

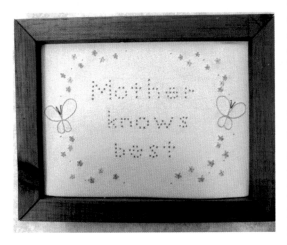

All this environmental talk comes down to, what should we be eating. Perhaps we have to admit that "mother knows best," or it might be "father knows best" as more fathers cook the family dinner. (My girls embroidered a saying and even made a frame for it. It says "mother knows best." It is one of my most-prized possessions and is hanging proudly in my bedroom.)

Eat your fruits and vegetables

Remember when your mother said to clean your plate? Perhaps those green, yellow and orange things were not your favorite. If you loved them as I did, you were one of the lucky ones. I learned to love the fresh vegetables from the large suburban garden grown by my dad. Since he spent hours poring over numbers as an accountant, gardening was his relaxation. He even enjoyed sitting on the back steps shelling peas and shucking corn. What we couldn't eat went into the freezer. The taste of those fresh vegetables was something special.

More and more research by nutritionists has shown the importance of consuming the vitamins, minerals, and the unseen micro-nutrients found in dark-colored vegetables and fruits.

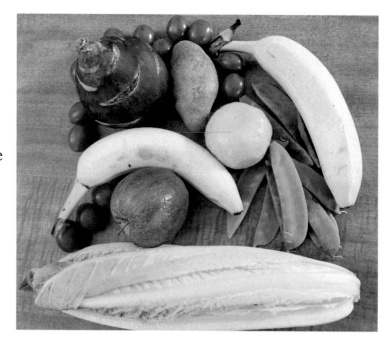

When I was studying for my nutrition degree at Syracuse University during the 70s, I clearly remember a guest speaker from Cornell University talking about his new research into the cancer-preventing qualities of cruciferous vegetables. These marvelous natural "drugs" are found particularly in broccoli, cauliflower, cabbage and Brussel sprouts. (Unfortunately, they are also known for producing intestinal gas - bring on the Beano.)

Colors are good

What other vegetables are especially good? High in beta-carotene which becomes Vitamin A in the body are carrots, sweet potatoes, pumpkin, butternut squash, (yellow is the key) also spinach, kale and red peppers. They are good for normal vision (helping to prevent macular degeneration), strengthening the immune system, and reproduction. The animal sources are egg yolk (note that it is yellow) and cheddar cheese. (1)

B-complex vitamins are complex because this is the overall name for: thiamine (B1), riboflavin (B2), niacin (B3), pantothenic acid (B5), pyridoxine (B6), biotin (B7), folate (B9) and cobalamin (B12). Again, color is good since dark green leafy vegetables are good sources of folate and other B vitamins.

One caveat regarding greens – be sure you wash them well. Romaine lettuce has been under scrutiny because some was contaminated during the growing and/or processing. Usually the problem is that feedlots for animals are too close to the growing fields and the manure seeps into the water source for irrigation of the crops. Most of the greens are grown in Salinas Valley and other parts of California as well as Arizona. The culprit is mostly E. coli which can cause severe kidney problems. The incidence is fairly rare, but caused the recall of all Romaine lettuce from some growers in California in October – December 2019. More inspections are needed.

A report in *Consumer Reports* in March 2020 suggested washing your lettuce in a vinegar bath. It should be refrigerated and used soon after purchase. The best bet is organic or leafy greens grown in a greenhouse or hydroponically. It is better to buy a whole head rather than the packaged variety because there is less chance of contamination during the processing. (2)

Kermit the Frog was right

It may not be easy being green, but eating green is easy. Overall, leafy greens are a good thing to eat. Iceberg lettuce is unfortunately low on the list of nutrient-dense greens. Kale is good for preventing macular degeneration (a condition of the eyes that prevented my dad from pursuing his many hobbies in his 90s) and possibly cataracts. Romaine is good for vitamin A and folate, and is a favorite for its crispness. Spinach has vitamin K, potassium and folate, but is best cooked to break down the oxalic acid to make the calcium and iron it contains available to the body.

Legumes are also good sources of folate (B9) and include kidney beans, edamame, soy nuts and peas. Some fish are good sources especially of B12 and include oysters, clams and mussels. Animal sources such as milk (B2) eggs (B7), yogurt (B12), chicken and turkey (B3) are also good for B vitamin content. Sunflower seeds which provide 20% of B5 per ounce are another source.

Valentine red for a healthy heart

Tomatoes are a good choice, especially when cooked. They are high in lycopene, which has been linked to many health benefits, including reduced risk of heart disease and cancer. They are a great source of vitamin C, potassium, folate and vitamin K. (3)

Vitamin C is important for maintaining good health, though the idea that it prevents a cold has been disproved. It is a delicate vitamin and doesn't like heat or light. Vitamin C is found in citrus food like oranges, strawberries, kiwi fruit, bell peppers, broccoli, kale and spinach.

Vitamin D is rightly named the sunshine vitamin. That means that we have a substance in our bodies that makes it from sunshine. If you live in a gloomy state such as in the Northeast where I live, you probably don't get enough. Some sources are salmon, trout and egg yolks. Vitamin D is added to milk and dairy products, but you may need to take a pill to supplement your diet. However, it is stored in the body, so don't overdo.

Seniors beware

Older adults may be lacking in certain essential nutrients. This is possibly because of medications they take, or because they have trouble absorbing and utilizing them. Vitamin B12 is an important vitamin which can be affected by acid controllers such as omeprazole, or by diabetes medications such as metformin. According to Joshua Miller, professor and chair of the department of nutritional sciences at Rutgers University, doctors are not always looking at B12 when people over 60 develop signs of deficiency such as fatigue, tingling in hands or feet, or irritability, among other symptoms. (4)

Good sources of B12 are animal products including dairy, fish, and eggs. Vegetarians and vegans may be lacking in B12. Getting tested for this is a good idea, and may require supplementation. (5)

The egg and I

Eggs are excellent sources of protein and vitamins. However, a recent study done at Northwestern University showed that three or more eggs per week increased the chance of a *17 percent higher risk of incident cardiovascular disease and 18 percent higher risk of deaths from all causes.* The problem with the study is that it was based on a short time-frame and relied on food recall by the participants. The jury is still out, but it might be wise to limit your consumption of eggs. As always, moderation is the key. (6) Though full of cholesterol, they are now thought not to be as great a problem as once believed.

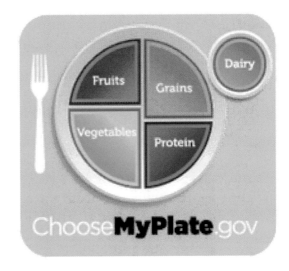

Get your fiber

We can take multi-vitamin tablets, but we don't get those micro-nutrients which are still being discovered. More importantly, they don't include fiber. Fiber is another essential in our diet which is found especially in the skins of vegetables and fruits. In many cases, you

This revised suggestion for a dinner plate includes one-half devoted to fruits and vegetables and only one-quarter to a protein and one-quarter to a whole grain.

don't need to remove the skin from potatoes or carrots. There are healthy nutrients just under the skin. Hamburgers and French fries provide fat and calories, but little fiber.

Fill your plate wisely

The current idea is to rethink a healthy plate with less emphasis on protein, otherwise known as the entree, and more emphasis on the accompanying vegetables and fruits, as well as whole grains. The healthy plate has one-quarter protein, one-quarter whole grain and one-half vegetables and/or fruit.

The more I read about the impact of food on the environment and climate change, the more I recognize the intersection of good nutrition and a healthy earth. Dr. Walter C. Willett agrees. He is professor emeritus of epidemiology and nutrition at Harvard's T. H. Chan School of Public Health as well as professor of medicine at Harvard Medical School, and author of 1800 studies.

Dr. Willett calls his diet the "flexitarian diet." The basis of the diet is plants. Only a very small amount, about one-half an ounce a day, of red meat. That means once a month you might have a steak. As explained in an earlier chapter, cows produce methane, a potent greenhouse gas, and also breathe out carbon dioxide. Beef cows take several years of consuming grass to be ready for slaughter, all the while consuming precious water and usually grain. (7)

He unequivocally states, "we simply cannot eat the amounts of beef that we're now consuming and still have a future for our grandchildren." (7) From a nutritional standpoint, beef has a large amount of saturated fat - that marbling that makes the meat tender. This is not a good thing for our level of cholesterol, and bad for our hearts.

On the other hand, according to Dr. Willett, pigs are ready for market in six months and will eat scraps, thus are not as big a problem. Chickens are ready in six weeks and don't have time to produce as much "bad breath" as cows.

As mentioned in Chapter six, fish are great for our diet, but over-fishing and warmer oceans are making fish consumption a luxury. As mentioned in Chapter six, more work needs to be done on farming fish in ponds that are regularly cleaned, especially those imported from other countries.

Protein comes in many forms

In our red-meat culture, we tend to forget that there are many other sources of protein. Other sources are actually less expensive and very nutritious such as beans, soy, tempeh, tofu and various kinds of nuts.

Walnuts are especially good sources of omega-3s and high in anti-oxidant properties. A single serving of one ounce (10 -12 whole walnuts or 1/4 cup) provides a day's supply of the good type of fat. According to Registered Dietitian Marsha McColloch, walnuts also fightinflammation, and promote the healthy bacteria in the intestines. She suggests that they help lower the risk of colon cancer and help lower blood pressure And because they contain: *polyunsaturated fat, polyphenols and vitamin E,* she suggests that they may be helpful for your brain function. That is quite a load for those little nuts to carry. They also carry a hefty calorie count of 190 calories per serving, but in moderation are well worth it. (8)

If you have diabetes, nuts have an even greater benefit in cutting heart disease. A long-term study reported in *Circulation* showed that eating *"about a quarter cup of nuts five times or more a week cut their risk for coronary heart disease by 20 percent as compared with those who eat nuts less than once per month."* (9)

There are other nuts that provide similar benefits. These include: almonds, pistachios, pecans, cashews and Brazil nuts. Macadamia nuts contain mono-unsaturated fats, the good kind of fat. Peanuts are also good, though they are not technically a tree nut, but are rather in the legume family. Peanut butter is an excellent source, but choose the kind without added sugar and lower in salt content. (10)

Bread is the staff of life

According to Dr. Willett, in the U.S. 45% of grain is used to feed animals, 30% goes to ethanol, and 15 % to high-fructose corn syrup. Only 10% is used to feed us. Since we are hopefully vowing not to waste grain on feeding beef cattle, we can be more choosey about the grain we feed ourselves. (11)

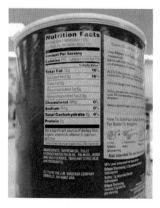

Grain is an important part of a human healthy diet. However, not just any old grain is best. Whole grain, the part that includes the outer coat of bran is much more nutritious and adds to our fiber needs. Choosing not only whole-grain bread, but whole-grain pizza crust, whole-grain pasta and even whole-grain cereal is possible. It even has more flavor than the boring white-wheat stuff.

Trans-fat has fortunately been eliminated thanks to the Center for Science in the Public Interest. This canned fat is not as bad as it once was, but liquid fat is better.

Good fats versus bad fats

We hear so much about bad fat, and low-fat diets. However, fat is an essential part of our diet. Cholesterol is a building block of our cells, and thus it is not all bad. Our body can produce most of the fat it needs, but not all. The important thing is choosing the right fats.

The worst offender is **trans-fat**. This is totally unnatural fat, made by a chemical manufacturing process. Unfortunately, though nutrition labels must show trans-fat content, if it is under 1%, it can count as zero. It is known to be very bad for your heart. If you see the words partially-hydrogenated fat, that is trans-fat. Technically it means that hydrogen atoms have been added to change the fat from liquid to solid.

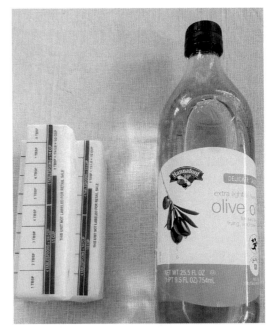

Choose olive oil instead of butter. The oil has monounsaturated fat and is a feature of the Mediterranean diet. Butter is tasty but high in saturated fat.

Remember those cans of shortening which we used to make really flaky pie crust? We used to call them "fat in a can." That is a can full of trans-fat and not available in my household. The *Center for Science in the Public Interest* was successful in getting trans-fat banned from food through extensive lobbying of Congress.

Another offender is saturated fat. That is the one found especially in red meat and full-fat dairy. It tends to be one that clogs your arteries and increases LDL (the bad cholesterol) in your blood. (11)

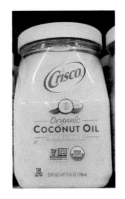

Coconut oil is also high in saturated fat. Though olive oil is the best fat, it not good at high termperatures. Canola oil is good for frying

On blood tests you will see a number for LDL or low-density lipoproteins.   These are the ones that cling to the arteries and cause a build-up of plaque - not a good thing. When the arteries narrow, blood flow is restricted - high blood pressure and heart problems can be the result.

To counteract that, you will see a number for the good fat, HDL (high density lipoprotein). This is the one that keeps the fat moving so that it doesn't cling to your arteries and cause a problem. A high number here is a good sign. It can be a sign that you eat well and get lots of exercise. Unfortunately, it is not the whole answer. Some problems with cholesterol can be genetic and may require a prescription drug.

An example of a good fat is a polyunsaturated fat. This means liquid fat and includes such things as canola oil, soy oil, and vegetable oil.

Very good fats are mono-unsaturated fats. The best example is olive oil. You often hear about the merits of the Mediterranean diet. Those dishes often include olive oil. (12)

What is on the bad food list?

Just like Santa has a list of bad behavior, food scientists in their white lab coats have a list of bad foods. Pure sugar probably tops the list because it provides only calories. Naturally we can splurge sometimes, but here again, moderation wins. Sugar comes in many forms and manufacturers like to fool you with different names: dextrose, sucrose, fructose, high-fructose corn syrup, etc.

There are all kinds of additives on that bad list. This includes nitrates and nitrites. Luncheon meats and bacon often use these as a preservative. They are also found in most wine. The problem is that they convert to nitrites when cooked at high temperature and this is a known carcinogen. Is it worth a dose of cancer in your daily sandwich? Here again moderation is the key. You can now find some of these that advertise nitrate-free, but you have to read the labels.

Nitrate-free does not mean problem-free however. I recently learned that the celery liquid used in the nitrate-free products like hot dogs has the same effects in the body as do the nitrates. This is still a controversial topic. (13)

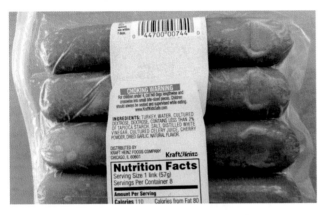

I like these turkey hot dogs because they are nitrate-free. However they have celery juice as a preservative, which may also be a carcinogen.

Dyes are another problem. All they provide is color, and can cause allergies. (I have that problem.) Look for natural dyes like turmeric.

Train yourself to read labels. It makes a trip to the grocery store more time-intensive. But after a while you will know the best foods to buy.

Can't pronounce it, don't eat it

Read the ingredient list on many things that we eat today and much is unpronounceable. It was a surprise to me to learn that we should thank the military for many of these "improvements" in our diet. The saying that *an army marches on its stomach* is so true.

According to Anastacia Marx de Salcedo in her book *Combat-Ready Kitchen,* many of the easy meals and snacks we eat today were developed in laboratories supported by the military in the important effort to develop foods that are stable in many environments, easily transported over many miles, light-weight, and yes, even edible. Without the last essential point, most of these foods would fill garbage dumps and not provide the energy for soldiers to march, point and shoot. (14)

The hardtack of the Civil War was exactly that, hard and very chewy. Without methods of refrigeration, pre-food known as "beef on the hoof," and made from a variety of animals followed the armies to battle. Without provisions, starvation and disease, plus looting of farms and homes, were major problems.

With the invention of the can, canned meat was used in subsequent wars. Storage, weight, and shelf-life were all problems to be overcome, not to mention that pesky taste problem.

Later, meat-packing plants in Chicago developed methods of deboning the beef carcass in obnoxious ways that we probably don't want to know about. Still today, nobody wants a meat-processing plant in their backyard. (An area just south of where I live was successful in fighting one.)

Restructured meat was the result of the food scientists at the Department of Defense supported laboratories such as the Natick Center in Massachusetts experimenting with different methods of making pseudo-meat taste like the real thing. It also had to be free of bacteria, molds and other disease-promoting entities. Hence, we see various chemical preservatives appear in these meat products. (14)

Here packaging methods also enter the picture, with the military using vacuum-packed foil and plastic packets to help with the storage issues. These are lighter, and can be stacked in trucks or backpacks. However, elements in the plastic can leach into the food, and this hasn't been studied adequately.

All these things osmosed into the consumer market. And an entire case at the supermarket is filled with various sandwich meats - which means a quick sandwich can be made with a square "just the right size" as a slice of bread.

Also notice the list of preservatives, especially note nitrites which were discussed above.

However, those of you who read Chapter five, know that eating red meat is not a good thing, so hopefully you will fill your grocery cart with other options.

In addition to food, of course we also need lots of liquids. There is much from which to choose.

How sweet it is

Soda has become the beverage of choice for many. Unfortunately it has replaced milk in the diets of many growing children, not a good thing in terms of nutrition.

Regular cola contains a huge amount of sugar. One twelve ounce glass (bottle or can) has 10 1/4 teaspoons of sugar, and 150 kcal. No wonder it tastes so sweet. (15) It also has a significant amount of caffeine.

Sugar is usually something to be avoided because it lacks nutritional value and is high in calories. An option for many of us are artificial sweeteners, especially for anyone with diabetes or who is on a diet. They also do not promote tooth decay.

Thus many have turned to diet soda. It lacks calories but the sweetness comes from one of a variety of artificial ingredients.

The safety of these is a concern, though the "jury is still out" on which is the best one to use. Perhaps you can be like my son-in-law and develop a dislike for anything sweet; however, that is rare. "But according to the National Cancer Institute and other health agencies, there's no sound scientific evidence that any of the artificial sweeteners approved for use in the United States cause cancer or other serious health problems" (16)

Stevia is an unusual case. It is considered "natural" because it is derived from a natural source. Much sweeter than sugar, it is derived from a bushy plant related to the sunflower. It is grown in Paraguay, Brazil, Japan and China, and thus all is imported.

From an environmental standpoint, it takes less land and water than other sweeteners. However, it does require bleaching and removing the color to take out the bitterness. (17)

Honey is also a natural product. It has some antibacterial properties. However, it should not be given to children under the age of one because it may contain "small amounts of bacterial spores that can produce botulism toxin." (18)

Molasses is also a sweetener featured in delicious cookies. Formed as a byproduct of the manufacture of sugar cane and sugar beets, it varies in color and intensity. It is generally thick and viscous, thus difficult to pour. Blackstrap is the most concentrated and also has the most vitamins and minerals, but is also rather bitter. Light molasses is most often used in baking and is more sweet. Sulphured molasses means that sulphur dioxide has been added as a preservative. Because it is high in carbohydrates, it is not recommended in large amounts. On the plus side, it contains manganese, magnesium, potassium and iron. (19)

Any sweetener with a name ending in "ol" is a sugar alcohol. This includes sorbitol and mannitol. These are somewhat less sweet than sugar, while many of the others are sweeter than sugar. The problem with sugar alcohol is that an excess amount can cause bloating and diarrhea.

Some artificial sweeteners have an aftertaste. The choice is personal preference. As with most foods, moderation is the key.

Elsie the cow gives us milk

Most of you are not old enough to remember Elsie the Cow. She was a popular advertising symbol for milk when I was young.

Milk is a controversial subject. Some people have lactose intolerance. This means that they cannot digest the milk sugar or lactose in milk and therefore must give up milk. Lactose-free

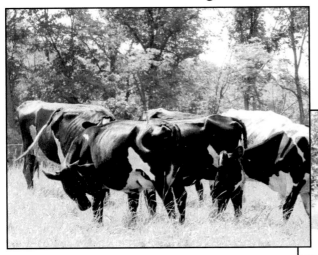

These cows produce organic milk for Organic Valley brand. They eat grass and roam freely. As you see, this organic farmer, Sarah Huftalen, is proud of her product.

milk is one alternative. There are many types of milk substitutes such as: almond milk, soy milk, oat milk and coconut milk. According to *Consumer Reports*, there has been a huge upswing in the use of plant-based milk in recent years. (20) A variety of reasons cause people to choose these: they cannot tolerate dairy products, they want to avoid animal products, or they think it is healthier.

The problem is that *"few of the drinks...tested match cow's milk for nutrition."* (20) Other milks often contain added sugar and chemical additives. The concern is the addition of tricalcium phosphate and disodium phosphate to stabilize the milk and to add calcium and phosphorus to try to match cow's milk in nutritional value. However, *"a high intake of these additives may increase the risk of kidney disease, heart disease, and bone loss."* (20) Carrageenan, a seaweed extract, is added to some almond milks and may *"trigger inflammation in people who suffer from colitis and other inflammatory bowel disorders."* (20)

Are they better for the planet? Yes and no. Water usage is a concern. Soy and oat milk score well, but almond milk uses a great deal of water. If you choose organic, it will reduce the problems caused by the use of pesticides; which is also true for cow's milk.

Thinking I had a problem, I gave up cow's milk for a long time, and it was painful since I love milk and ice cream. Now I do drink low-fat cow's milk because of taste and the nutritional value. You cannot beat it for natural amounts of protein, calcium, potassium and B vitamins, plus the Vitamin D added to most. I bribe my partner with some chocolate in his milk in order to get him to drink it – you do what you have to do.

Whole milk and cheese do have the problem of being high in saturated fat. Therefore, it is better to use low-fat or skim milk and mozzarella cheese made from part skim-milk. Children between weaning and two do need whole or 2% milk or a comparable substitute for good brain and bone development. (21)

Fruit juice has a juicy secret

Unfortunately, arsenic and lead have been found in fruit juice. Apple juice is one of the worst offenders, perhaps because of all the spraying of apple trees as mentioned in Chapter eight. Also, juice does not have much fiber, thus does not fill you up, especially if you are trying to lose weight. (22)

Surprisingly, beer actually has helpful nutrients such as B vitamins. But don't overdo for obvious reasons. (23)

Caffeine is a mixed pleasure

Coffee has a lot of caffeine, tea has somewhat less and many soda drinks are high. There is a new craze - high-caffeine energy drinks. There is no doubt that caffeine can provide a boost of short-term energy. However, *the American Academy of Pediatrics* takes the position that *"stimulant-containing energy drinks have no place in the diets of children or adolescents."* The Mayo Clinic suggests that, *"if your caffeine habit totals more than 400 milligrams (mg) a day, you may want to consider cutting back."* (24) This is the amount in two to four 8-oz. cups.

Many folks find that coffee interrupts sleep if taken too late in the day. It can also irritate the stomach and cause jitters or migraines. (24)

On the plus side, it can fight inflammation in the body and contains some antioxidants. Decaffeinated coffee provides the same benefits. Coffee also may help dieting and may be good for brain health. There is even some evidence that it fights some types of cancer. (24)

The bitter pill is that we all need moderation in most things, food and drink being among them.

Tea for you

Another caffeinated beverage is tea, though it has less caffeine than coffee. (Tea has from 21 - 43 mg of caffeine per 100 g depending on brewing time. Brewed coffee has 104 mg/100 g and expresso from Starbucks has 250 mg/100 g. That will really wake you up.) (25)

All kinds of tea have benefits, though green tea has the most because of its larger supply of polyphenols. (Coffee also has these, though not in the quantity found in tea.) Polyphenols are antioxidants. They combine with oxidants which can cause harm, making them less likely to attack artery walls. Polyphenols also help reduce inflammation in the body. (26)

A number of large studies reported in the New York Times have shown a number of benefits of drinking tea. The problem with these studies is that is very difficult to prove cause and effect, and many studies were conducted in countries where tea is consumed in greater quantities than in the U.S. (27)

Some studies showed that *"tea was also associated with a reduction in the risk of stroke, with those consuming at least three cups a day having a 21 percent lower risk than those consuming less than a cup a day."* (27) This may because of those good polyphenols.

In other studies, tea has been associated with a reduction in various types of liver disease. There was also some reduction shown in the risk of developing type 2 diabetes. *"For each additional two cups per day of tea consumed, the risk of developing diabetes dropped 4.6 percent."* (27)

Tea does not appear to have any ill effects, except perhaps that when consumed in large quantities it can stain teeth. Ice tea is especially welcome in our increasingly hot climate. Thus it is probably a good idea to add tea to your list of beverages consumed.

Water wins the day

Water is still the best drink overall. But the pricey *special waters* provide no benefit. From an environmental standpoint, please forgo those plastic bottles unless your water has been contaminated. Tap water must be inspected if it comes from a municipal source and is usually safe. If you have a well, the water should have been tested when the well was installed. You can also have it tested at a local testing facility.

Bottled water is usually not tested extensively. Testing by the Food and Drug Administration which regulates bottled water has actually declined, and the budget of that department has been significantly cut back in recent years. One brand owned by Keurig Dr. Pepper had to be taken off the market because, unbelievably, it was found to contain arsenic. (28)

Obviously there have been major problems in municipal water systems, which have been widely reported in the media, such as Flint, Michigan and Newark, New Jersey. Several villages near where I live have also had major problems with their water supplies. Lead in the water due to aging pipes is also a concern.

In fact, U.S. citizens spent $31 billion on bottled water, thinking it is safer. This often is not the case. (29) The bottled water industry helps feed this concern because it aids their bottom line. According to Food and Water Watch, *"nearly 64 percent of bottled water sold in the U.S. is filtered tap water."* (30)

Two of the most popular brands of bottle water actually come from municipal sources. Dasani is owned by Coca-Cola and Aquafina is a Pepsi product. Poland Spring comes from underground supplies rather than an actual spring. It is owned by Nestlé (28) and is currently being sued because the water does not originate from water running from a spring, and is depleting the spring's water supply. To their credit, Poland Spring has a report on the content of their water on their website. (31)

Remember mention of Fuji water in Chapter seven (or haven't you been paying attention)? This is artesian water from an underground source accessed through a well. It travels several thousand miles from this South Pacific island to reach your table, and is Fiji's biggest export. (32) At least we are helping to keep their residents employed, and think of all the ship's captains and truck drivers getting paid. However, the cost to the environment is even higher.

From an environmental standpoint, water has a number of advantages. In most cases it is available locally. It does not require bottling and packaging.

Say no to antibiotics

Even the water we use to clean our hands is being contaminated, by antibiotics and anti-bacterial agents.

We are developing resistance to antibiotics because of their overuse. According to the Center for Disease Control, *"each year in the U.S., at least 2 million people are infected with antibiotic-resistant bacteria, and at least 23,000 people die as a result."* (33) They also state that nearly 20,000 people died in 2017 of deadly Staphylococcus aureus (better known as Staph) infections. Hospital-based infections can make going to the hospital "risky business."

Unfortunately, beef and poultry producers like them because antibiotics prevent and treat infections. Though this is controversial, part of the problem may be the way in which poultry producers are becoming larger operations with thousands of chickens crowded in small spaces.

Antibiotics also fatten beef, chickens and turkeys more quickly, getting them ready for market in record time. This means more profits for the producers.

A report on Frontline, a program on the Public Broadcasting System (PBS) stated that: *"concern about the growing level of drug-resistant bacteria has led to the banning of sub-therapeutic use of antibiotics in meat animals in many countries in the European Union and Canada."* (34) Tyson Foods, Perdue Farms and Foster Farms have pledged to eliminate antibiotics in feed. McDonald's and Wendy's have agreed to buy chicken raised without antibiotics. Lack of antibiotics is a good reason to buy organic poultry, though currently the cost is higher.

People requesting antibiotics from doctors is a huge part of the problem. Antibiotics are effective only for bacterial infections, not those caused by a virus. Sometimes doctors prescribe them even when they are not necessary because it makes patients think they are doing something. Always question if an antibiotic is needed. If you really need an antibiotic, you don't want to be resistant to its effects. (35)

Antibacterial is not needed

Avoiding antibacterial products is also an important rule to follow. According to the FDA, antibacterial soaps are no more effective in cleaning and preventing disease than plain old soap and water. They also have the potential to create bacteria that are resistant to antibiotics. Also, they could act as endocrine disruptors, interfering with thyroid function. (36)

In addition, they are bad for the environment. They contain triclosan, which gets flushed down the drain. Small quantities of this chemical can sneak through water treatment plants undetected. Triclosan can disrupt algae in streams and other bodies of water interrupting the photosynthesis process. (37) Another study in 2008 found triclosan in the urine of 75 percent of those studied. This is probably due to absorption through the skin, and perhaps ingestion.

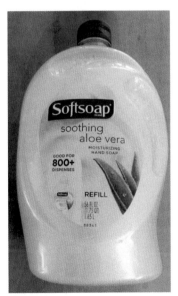

Many other products advertised as antibacterial include triclosan. These include: skin cleansers, deodorants, lotions, creams, toothpastes,

This liquid dish soap is made with einvironmentally friendly ingredients.

Soap without any antibacterial agents can be purchased in large bottles and used to refill the small pump bottles.

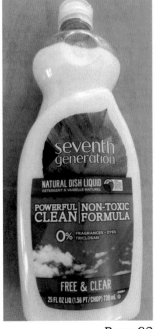

and dishwashing liquids and even fabrics. (38)

Finding liquid soap not labeled antibacterial is challenging, but not impossible. I keep a large bottle of plain liquid soap in my basement to refill my dispenser bottles. For the most part I rely on Dove soap in my soap dish. Remember to scrub for about 30 seconds, enough time to sing "Happy Birthday to you" twice.

Hints

Avoid anti-bacterial products, especially soap
Don't buy food with added nitrates
Buy colorful fruits and vegetables, hopefully organic
Use good fats like olive oil
Eat eggs and drink coffee in moderation
Increase fiber in your diet
Consume nuts in small quantities for their good protein
Use water filters and refillable bottles, not plastic bottles.

Chapter eleven
Grocery Shopping

We are such spendthrifts with our lives, the trick of living is to slip on and off the planet with the least fuss you can muster. I'm not running for sainthood. I just happen to think that in life we need to be a little like the farmer, who puts back into the soil what he takes out.
— Paul Newman

Some folks love shopping in the supermarket, some hate it. It can either be an excursion, and time to delight in all the choices available, perhaps seeing friends and neighbors. Or it can mean too many difficult choices and decisions, and time taken from hobbies. I tend to fall in the latter category.

Hopefully you have become a label reader. That definitely takes more time and dedication, as well as the reading glasses. A recent push by the *Center for Science in the Public Interest* has made many labels larger and more legible. However, once you get in a pattern of buying only healthy products and those with fewer additives, it becomes easier. Advice usually given is to concentrate on the outside edges of the store where lies the produce and less adulterated foods. Usually you know what you can actually get your family to eat, with a few excursions into something more daring. Less processing is generally better.

In the best of all worlds, you have shopped at a farmer's market or purchased a share in a CSA (Community Supported Agriculture). Perhaps the weather has allowed you to grow your own vegetables in the backyard, or in a container on your patio or balcony.

Food

Transportation costs

It is always better to buy items which are made close to home. This is where it gets tricky. Do you buy the healthier choice, or the one grown locally? You want your Vitamin C from fresh oranges, or your potassium from bananas, but they come all the way from another state or country. In terms of the environment, which is hopefully our big concern, the fossil fuel used in transporting that food over long distances is a crime. It is a tough choice, however, I usually the tip the balance toward what is most healthy for my family.

Why does organic matter?

The biggest difference between organic and industrial-produced food is the use of pesticides and fertilizer on the latter. Poisons get

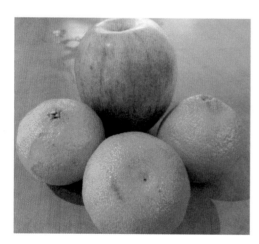

in the food, and it does not wash off easily. Especially with food in which we eat the skin, this is a major concern. Fruits and vegetables such as strawberries, spinach, kale, grapes and tomatoes (which are actually a fruit) are better if organic. I can't deny that organic costs more. If only growers understood how much more they could make by growing crops using organic or sustainable methods. We need to encourage more growers to practice sustainable farming. (1) (2)

No matter what produce you buy, **always wash it,** even if it has a tough skin. Examples are oranges, bananas and avocado. There have been cases of poison found on the skin of this produce forcing a recall. Always wash everything you eat!

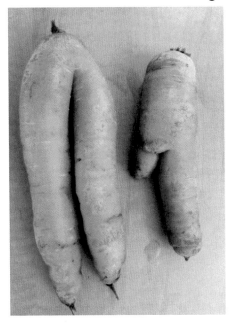

These ugly carrots taste just as good. Just cut off any bad parts and cook. This ugly beet will also make a tasty dish.

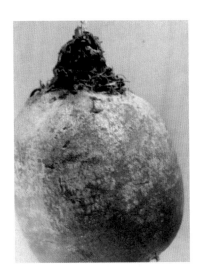

Produce doesn't have to be model perfect

There are some companies now that will sell you produce that is not perfect. So much ends up in the recycling bin. Online companies such as Imperfect Produce and Hungry Harvest will actually deliver this to your door and they advertise that their products cost less than the supermarket. Hungry Harvest is limited to certain states in the Northeast. (3) Imperfect Produce is based in San Francisco and delivers on the west coast. Walmart is also getting into this market.

As reported in the Washington Post, *The United States throws away tons of edible food every year.* This amounts to 63 million tons of waste a year, and the waste of 21% of all the fresh water in the country. It contributes to 21% of the land fill. (4)

Skip the bottled water, juice and bottled coffee

As discussed in Chapter ten, a full 47 percent of bottled water sold in the U.S. comes from tap water. A recent study comparing tap water and bottled water, showed that bottled water with more acidity may contribute to the demineralization and deterioration of teeth. Water that is treated with osmosis will be more acid. Low acidity (a low Ph) may contribute to other health problems as well. (5)

If you want an energy boost, stick to a brewed cup of coffee. An energy drink delivers about the same amount of caffeine as **four cups** of coffee, along with nearly 10 teaspoons of sugar and some non-FDA-approved ingredients. It may even lead to cardiac death and potentially dangerous changes in heartbeat and blood pressure. My significant other had to give up coffee altogether after he developed a blocked bundle-branch in his heart, due to excess caffeine.

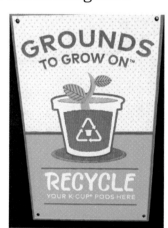

Personally, I am opposed to the pre-measured coffee pods for a number of reasons. Most important from an environmental standpoint is the fact that the paper cup adds substantially to our food waste. Additionally, it is much more expensive than buying a bag of beans. I have an inexpensive coffee grinder and it makes a better-tasting drink. You can also buy the already ground coffee if you plan to use it in a short time. Stopping at your local coffee bar adds substantially to the cost. Make your coffee the night before and heat in the microwave if you are in a hurry.

These small recycling containers will find reuses fo coffee pods. This one was found in the kitchen of a local church.

The present is plastics

The iconic phrase uttered 50 years ago in the movie, <u>The Graduate</u>, *"the future is plastics"* has become reality. Developed through testing sponsored by the military to ensure longevity of food for the troops, plastic is now very much a part of the shopping experience. From the plastic bags we are given to carry

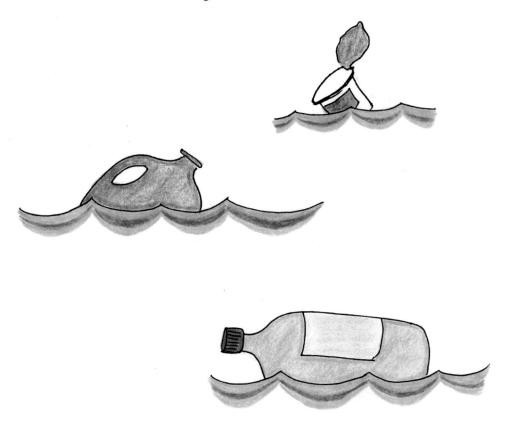

Plastics never disintegrate. Many end up polluting our oceans and are eaten by fish. They are ground up into tiny particles that become part of our food and even our toothpaste. Illustration by Susan Lee Reardon.

our purchases out of the store, to the shrink wrap on meat and poultry products, to the plastic-lined juice boxes and the plastic baby bottles we give our children, plastic is everywhere.

Unfortunately, it is known that plastic often leaches into food from the packaging. What is not known is how much, if any, harm it causes. Microwave cooking has made plastic even more useful in heating food, but most types of plastic are not appropriate. These supposed advances are all the result of research by the military on finding ways to transport, store, and cook food during times of conflict. To pay for all this in times of peace, companies have adopted the techniques and sold them to us, the consumers, as a good thing.

Food

When you are buying your poultry and fish you will find it is usually shrink-wrapped in plastic. If you have a friendly butcher, he or she will wrap it in brown paper like in days past. In an effort to save labor costs, the neighborhood butcher is becoming more rare

The packaging itself can also be a concern. The plastic can leach into the food. Also, cans are usually coated with bisphenol-A or BPA which prevents the acid in the food from attacking the can. Only a few companies have removed this chemical from their cans, and other countries such as Austria and China are questioning its use. (6)

Plastic is a product of that fossil fuel, oil. People don't think of this when they pick up all that plastic at the supermarket. Not only are we running out of oil, if not now, sometime in the near future, but fossil fuel impacts the earth in so many ways. The production of the plastic itself causes environmental problems. Then there is the problem of all the plastic that ends up in the trash and in the oceans. Fish ingest it and we end up with plastic in our stomachs. Plastic does not disintegrate for hundreds of years.

Also try to avoid cosmetics which contain micro beads of plastic. If you have plastic bags, at least take them back to the recycling bins found in most drug stores and supermarkets.

According to a report in CBSNews.com, *"Four companies - Coca Cola, Mars, Nestlé and Danone - produce six million tons of plastic waste every year."* The good news is that they *"plan to make these recyclable within six years."* (7)

Cloth saves the day

Invest in some cloth bags and take them to the supermarket and to other stores. Or if you are clever you can make your own.

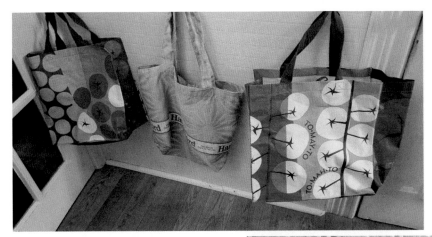

My reusable bags hang in my kitchen for easy access, and I keep some in my car.

The plastic wrap seen throughout the supermarket is avoided if you bring your own canvas, produce and other reusable bags. Keep some in your car. These are easily washed in the washing machine. Some states including New York State have eliminated the use of plastic bags, so cloth bags will become more common, Be ahead of the trend.

Reusable is key

Paper is not a good alternative. As mentioned previously, the process of making paper requires many unsavory chemicals. Avoid using paper plates and cups. Reusable is best. Also **avoid plastic and paper straws**.

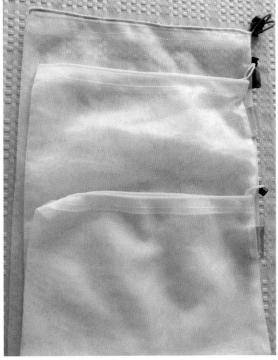

These are my produce bags, available on the internet. They are easily washed in the washing machine. I use them for my CSA vegetables, produce from the store, and even as a carry-on essentials for plane trips.

Food

They cause all kinds of problems in the ocean. Instead ask for your drink without ice, and you will not need a straw. There are also metal, reusable straws available.

When you eat out, bring your own take-out containers. Put half your entree in one to save calories and provide dinner another day. Most restaurant meals have grown to huge portions which provide much more than the body needs.

Penny wise and pound foolish

Buying organic and sustainably-grown foods is more expensive. However, there are ways to save. If you are eliminating red meat, you will save a significant amount. Buying from a farmer's market or a farm stand eliminates the middleman and is usually less expensive than the store. Planting your own garden is a great way to save. If you freeze the excess produce you will also be saving.

Cutting down on processed food is another way to save. Usually this is a healthier option. Snack foods are comforting, but usually not the best option from a health or financial standpoint. Also soda and bottled water are both expensive.

Cooking at home rather than eating at a restaurant or take-out saves a great deal of money. Usually homecooking can include more fruits and vegetables. It does take more time so that is a factor, because your time is also valuable.

The cost of health care can be factored into the equation. Paying for doctor visits and medication, as well as lost time from work because of poor nutrition can be very expensive.

During the current economic crisis, every penny counts. If you live in a "food desert" without as many choices it is a problem. However, if you are able to choose, buying food that is high in nutrition but perhaps not as much "fun" can actually save money.

Sally West Carman

You are voting with your wallet.

Hints

Buy organic if possible
Avoid processed food
Don't buy food preserved with nitrites
Use glass containers
Take cloth bags to the store
Avoid paper products
No more straws

Food

Chapter twelve
Recipes for a healthy future

Pan for success, not gold

Choose your pans wisely, especially frying pans. Teflon-coated pans, though easily cleaned, give off a chemical which is bad for the lungs. Remember the canary in the coal mine – it was used to warn miners of dangerous fumes in the mine. When I was cooking with my Teflon pan my grandson had to move his bird to an upstairs bedroom. That experience encouraged me to buy ceramic frying pans. Cast iron pans are excellent and actually put some useful iron in your diet when cooking anything acidic such as tomatoes. However, the downside is that they are heavy and difficult to clean.

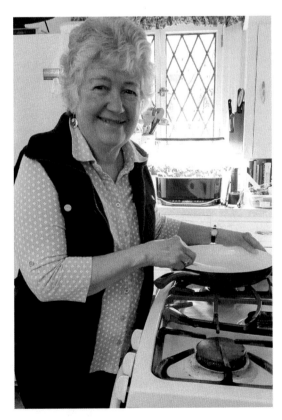

Here I am pretending to cook with my ceramic frying pan on my much-loved gas range.

Stainless steel pans are easily cleaned but do not transfer heat well, usually have a copper bottom or heat-transferring core is added. A pan that is flat on the bottom will conduct the heat from the range more readily, especially when

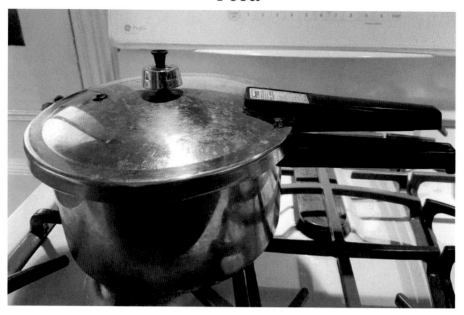

My sixty-year-old pressure cooker works well. The gasket has been the only thing replaced.

using a flat, top surface. Aluminum is an excellent conductor of heat, and the temporary concern that it would lead to Alzheimer's Disease has been thoroughly disproven (despite what the pot and pan salesmen try to tell you).

I have the same stainless-steel pans that I bought new in 1959 when I married. They still cook as well as ever, so they are long lasting. (Thanks go to the sorority sister who sold them to me.)

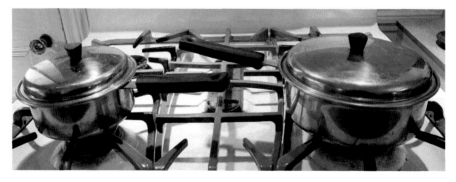

These stainless steel pans have also lasted for sixty years. Even the handles are still in good condition. (I like old and useful objects, like me.)

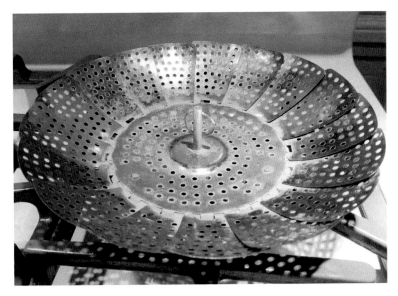

Consider a pressure cooker. I also have the same one I started married life with and it works fine. There are some new ones on the market and they have become popular again. It is great for making

This steaming rack can be used in a small pan to steam vegetables.

anything tender, and speeds up cooking time tremendously.

A steaming rack is also useful. Put it in the bottom of your pan when cooking vegetables with a small amount of water. It helps preserve the vitamins and minerals. However, you need to make sure the water does not run dry, as I have had that happen more than once.

I have not yet tried those frying machines. Always on a diet and concerned about too much fat, I try to avoid fried food.

A crock pot is a great way to save time late in the day. Start it early and dinner is ready when you get home from work or play.

Microwaves are great time savers. However, do not use any plastics in the microwave because there is a danger of chemicals from the plastics leaching into the food. Instead use ceramic or glass containers or microwaveable tableware such as plates and mugs.

Safety is always a concern, or should be. Never leave food out of

the refrigerator for more than two hours. If the container is still somewhat hot, put a pad under it in the refrigerator. Look for the "use by" date on the package. The "sell by" date does not indicate when the item must be cooked. When you see a "best by" date, it only indicates quality, not safety of the food
.

Soak your pans immediately after use – they will be much easier to wash. When using a dishwasher, be sure it is full before running it to save water and detergent. Also, please shut off the dry cycle; instead open the door when the washer finishes and air dry. I have very hard water in my village, and thus I have learned to put vinegar in the bottom of the dishwasher when I add the detergent. No extra chemicals are needed and it takes off all the film that collects on the glasses.

You don't have to be a great chef to make healthy meals. There are many quick meals that do not involve using processed foods. Some of the following recipes are easy and some more difficult. Don't hesitate to experiment a bit and change ingredients to suit your own allergies and tastes, and those of your family.

As Julia Child used to say, "Bon Appetit."

Soup

Chicken rice soup with vegetables
(1 serving. Multiply by number needed)

1 Tbsp concentrated chicken bouillon per serving
½ c instant brown rice
handful of washed organic spinach
½ c frozen peas
1½ c water

Heat in saucepan or microwave until it comes to a boil, reduce heat, cover and simmer for five minutes.
                    -Sally Carman

Carrot Vichyssoise

2 c   peeled, diced potatoes
¼ c   sliced organic carrots
3 c   chicken or vegetable broth
1 tsp   salt
1 c   2 % milk

Combine all ingredients in a saucepan, bring to a boil and simmer about 25 minutes until vegetables are tender. Cool, then puree in batches in a blender. Stir in the salt and then the milk. Serve hot or cold, garnished with parsley.

Food

Corn rice soup

1 can creamed corn
1 small pkg. frozen corn
1 container microwave pre-cooked
brown rice and quinoa
dried parsley flakes

Mix all together and add milk to
desired consistency. Heat to just
before boiling. Serve.

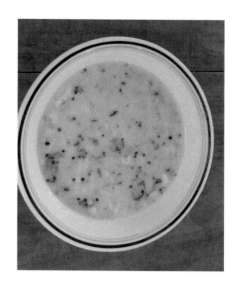

Minute vegetable soup

3 c water
2 c vegetables, grated (carrots, zucchini, celery, turnip or whatever
is on hand)
2 c chopped greens (spinach, celery, romaine lettuce, etc.)
½ c fine egg noodles or pasta
½ c parsley chopped
2 Tbsp melted butter

Boil water in a large saucepan. Grate and chop vegetables, add
to boiling water bring to another
boil, boil for five minutes.

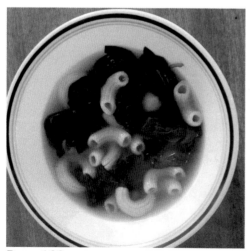

Vegan Soup

¼ onion chopped
1 yam chopped
1 white sweet potato chopped
2 celery stalks chopped
2 carrots chopped
½ tsp turmeric
1½ c cashew milk
1½ c vegetable broth
1 c frozen peas
¼ c nutritional yeast
2 cloves crushed garlic.
Salt and pepper

Add onion, garlic, yam, sweet potato, celery and carrots to a pot with enough vegetable stock to coat the bottom of the pan. Sweat the veggies on medium heat for 6 minutes stirring occasionally.

Add approximately 1 cup water and 1 cup vegetable broth to cover veggies. Bring to a boil and cover for 10 minutes.

Add frozen peas and reduce to simmer. Cover for 20 minutes

Add ½ teaspoon turmeric, 1½ cup cashew milk, and ¼ cup nutritional yeast. Add salt and pepper to taste and stir well. Simmer 5 minutes before serving

-Clifton Anderson

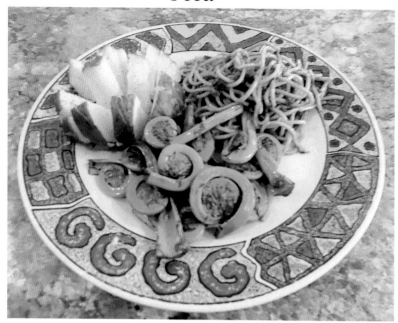

Main Dishes

Fiddleheads with sesame noodles

1/3 c.   sesame oil
1/3 c.   black soy sauce
1 ½   Tbsp. Black Chinese vinegar
2 Tbsp Hot pepper oil (or chili garlic sauce)
1   large bunch scallions or garlic chives
3 heaping Tbsp
            peanut butter

Mix these together and pour over:
1 lb.   cooked noodles
Refrigerate for 24 hours.
Wash fiddleheads well. (Fiddleheads can usually be picked the last week of April until the second week of May, depending on weather.)
Steam for 5 minutes, then sauté in olive oil and garlic for 5 minutes. Add seasoning to taste. Serve hot.
            -Dave Jones

Arizona Skillet Dinner

2 Tbsp	corn or canola oil
1 medium	onion, chopped
1 medium	green pepper, chopped
2 cloves	garlic, minced
2 tsp	chili powder
½ tsp	salt
½ tsp	ground cumin
1 can (28 oz)	crushed tomatoes
1 can (16oz)	kidney beans, rinsed & drained
1 pkg (10oz)	frozen corn kernels (thawed)
8 oz.	elbow macaroni, cooked, drained (about 1 3/4 cups cooked)
½ c	Shredded Monterey Jack Cheese with Jalapeno pepper (or plain)

In large skillet heat oil over medium-high heat. Add onion, green pepper, chili powder, salt and cumin; sauté 4 minutes or until vegetables are tender.

Stir in tomatoes. Add kidney beans and corn; bring to boil. Reduce heat and simmer 15 minutes, stirring occasionally. Toss with elbow macaroni.

Sprinkle with cheese. Makes 8 servings.

-Pam Fisher

Vegetable Pot Pie

Filling
2 medium-sized Portobello mushrooms
1 small sweet potato diced
1 large russet potato diced
¾ c frozen peas
2 carrots diced
3 Tbsp butter
3 Tbsp flour
1 tsp salt
1 tsp pepper
1 c vegetable stock
1 bouillon cube
1 c milk
2 Tbsp vegetable oil

Crust
2 c flour
2/3 c shortening
½ tsp salt
Ice-cold water

Place mixing bowl, spoon, and bowl of ice water in freezer ~20 min
Remove items from freezer, and stir together 2 cups flour and 1/2
tsp salt in chilled mixing bowl. Cut in shortening using a pastry
blender until pieces are pea-size. Pour in water 1 tablespoon
at a time, tossing moistened mixture, and pressing to the side
of the bowl. Repeat until entire mixture is moistened. Use the
minimum amount of water necessary. Divide in half and reserve
for later step.

Preheat oven to 350F

Heat vegetable oil in a large frying pan over medium heat. When
oil is hot, add Portabellas cap side up. Cook 3 minutes, flip,
and cook 3 more minutes. While mushrooms are cooking, dice
potatoes, sweet potato and carrots and boil in a small sauce pan

until fork tender (about 15 minutes). When Portabellas are done, place them on a cutting board to cool.

Rinse medium sauce pan and add butter, cooking on low heat. While butter is melting, measure out vegetable stock and milk and set aside. Warm the vegetable stock and place bouillon cube in the stock to dissolve. When the butter is melted add the flour. Cook 3 minutes stirring constantly. Whisk in vegetable stock until smooth. Whisk in 1 cup milk and let simmer, whisking frequently for 10 minutes. Reduce to very low heat. Add the frozen peas to a colander and pour the small sauce pan with potatoes and carrots over the peas allowing the hot water to drain.

Dice and add Portabellas and vegetables to sauce and stir. Roll out one of the pie crusts and place in a 10 in. deep-dish pie plate. Pour sauce into the crust and roll out second crust. Place the second crust on top of the filling and crimp the edges with a fork. Using a sharp knife, remove excess dough from the edge of the pie plate and cut slits in the top of the crust for venting. Bake 45 minutes (350 F). Remove from oven and cool for 15 min.

> - *Clifton Anderson*

Ratatouille Spaghetti

Vegetables:
Half of a large eggplant
3 Roma tomatoes
2 small zucchinis (green)
1 yellow squash
1 yellow bell pepper
1 red bell pepper
1 yellow onion
2 cloves of garlic

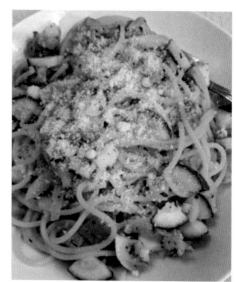

Seasonings: Salt, Pepper, Basil,
Parsley, Crushed red pepper,
Thyme
Extra virgin olive oil, grated parmesan cheese, 1 box of spaghetti

Bring a pot of salted water to boil. While water is heating, dice eggplant, tomatoes, zucchini, squash, bell pepper, and onion into similar-sized small pieces (approximately penny-sized or smaller). Crush and chop garlic.

Heat enough olive oil to coat the bottom of a large non-stick cooking pan on low-medium heat. Once oil is heated for approximately 1 minute, add garlic, onion and bell peppers to the pan. Stir frequently to start cooking, continuing with low-medium heat. After onion is beginning to turn translucent, add zucchini and squash to the pan. Add salt, pepper, and crushed red pepper to taste. You may need more salt that anticipated.

Begin cooking pasta- most spaghetti takes around 10 minutes. While pasta is cooking, add tomatoes and eggplant to the pan. Continue to cook the vegetable mixture and stir frequently on low-medium heat. Add basil, parsley, and thyme to taste. If preparing this recipe with dried spices, use a few extra dashes.
Add approximately 1 tablespoon of parmesan cheese to the pan with vegetables when pasta is almost done cooking. As pasta is nearly finished cooking, use tongs to grab pasta from the pasta

pot and add to the pan of vegetables. Continue mixing and cooking the pasta with the vegetables in the pan and reduce to a low heat. You can also add a few spoonsful of the water that the pasta boiled in the pan to increase moisture for the dish. After the vegetables and pasta are mixed thoroughly, serve with additional grated parmesan and a spoonful of olive oil.
-Rachel Franceschino

One-Pan Mexican Quinoa

4 servings
Prep time: 10 mins
Cook time: 25 min

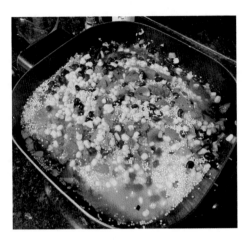

1 Tbsp olive oil
2 cloves garlic, minced
1 fresh jalapeno, minced
1 c quinoa
1 c vegetable broth
1 (15 oz) can black beans, drained and rinsed
1 (14.5 oz) can fire-roasted diced tomatoes

1 c corn kernels
1 tsp chili powder
½ tsp cumin
Salt and pepper, to taste
1 avocado, peeled and diced
1 lime or 2 Tbsp lime juice
2 Tbsp fresh chopped cilantro leaves

Heat olive oil in large skillet over medium high heat. Add garlic and jalapeno and cook, stirring frequently until fragrant, about 1 minute. Mix in quinoa, broth, drained beans, tomatoes, corn chili powder and cumin. Season to taste with salt and pepper. Bring to boil, cover and reduce heat to simmer for about 20 minutes, until quinoa is cooked through.
Remove from heat and stir in avocado, lime juice, and cilantro. Serve immediately. *-Sarah Koontz*

Chicken stir fry

8 oz. – 1 lb organic,
skin-free, chicken
Organic celery stalks
Roasted chestnuts
(optional)
Organic cherry
tomatoes
Can water chestnuts
Fresh pea pods
Organic soy sauce
Onion powder

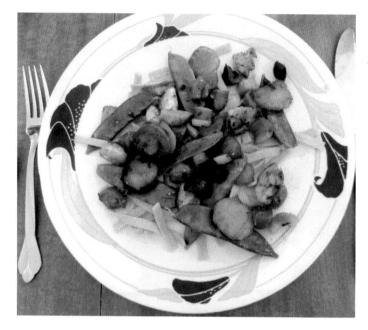

Heat canola oil in a
wok or frying pan.
Cut up chicken
into small bite-size
pieces, amount
dependent on
number of servings needed. Turn until evenly browned. Add
well-washed celery cut into small pieces. Sprinkle with soy sauce
and onion power to taste. Cover while preparing other ingredients.
Drain one can of water chestnuts, rinse and add to pan. Wash
cherry tomatoes and pea pods. Cut tomatoes in half. Add to pan
and stir. Add washed pea pods last and heat. Serve hot over
whole-wheat noodles.
        -Sally Carman

Turkey Meatloaf

2 lb.   ground turkey
2 pkg instant oatmeal, plain
1 c   1% milk
1   egg
2 Tbsp soy sauce
1½ tsp salt

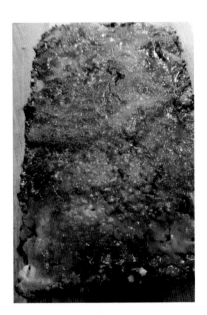

Mix all ingredients thoroughly and press into a loaf pan. Bake at 375 degrees for 75 minutes.

-Sally Carman

Turkey meatloaf two

1 lb.   ground turkey
2 Tbsp onion soup mix
1 small can condense milk

Mix all ingredients thoroughly and press into a loaf pan.

Top with:

2 Tbsp   catsup
2 Tbsp   Dijon mustard
2 Tbsp   brown sugar

Mix and spread on top.
Bake at 350 degrees for 45 minutes.

- C.A.W.

Vegetarian Spaghetti Sauce

To a crock pot add;
1 large can tomatoes
1 small can tomato sauce
(or substitute fresh tomatoes)
2 Tbsp quinoa
1 Tbsp salt
1 Tbsp onion powder
1 Tbsp basil
1 Tbsp dried parsley
1 Tbsp sugar (or Splenda)
1 tsp   oregano (or spices to taste)

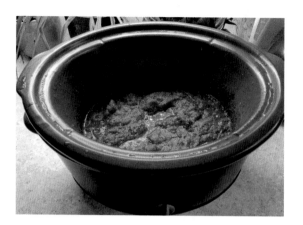

Add to crock pot. Cook on high for 4 hours and serve with cooked, whole-wheat spaghetti.
        -Sally Carman

Crockpot orange chicken

Mix 1 Tbsp chicken bouillon with water and place in crockpot
Add 2-3 boneless organic chicken breasts
Add thin skin small potatoes that have been scrubbed

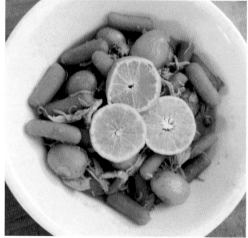

Wash organic carrots and add

Cook on high for 3 hours. Remove chicken and cut into small pieces.
Mix in 2 Tbsp soy sauce and 1/3 cup orange marmalade (made without sugar).

Cook for 1 more hour. Put into serving dish.
Garnish with orange slices and serve.   -Sally Carman

Chicken and biscuits

Fry two large chicken breasts in bottom of a pressure cooker.
Add 1 c. chicken bouillon
Add cut up organic carrots and
fingering potatoes, both washed carefully
Season with 2 Tbsp of soy sauce
Cook under pressure for 12 minutes.
(This may be served now and reheat as below.)

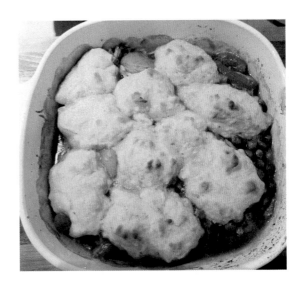

Transfer to a baking dish.
Combine 2 c. baking mix with 2/3 c. milk
Drop by tablespoons on top of chicken dish.
Bake at 375 degrees for 20 minutes.

-Sally Carman

Almond-crusted chicken

¼ c   sliced almonds
½ c   allpurpose flour
1 tsp   dry thyme
1 tsp   onion powder
1 tsp   garlic powder
½ tsp   salt
½ tsp   pepper
½ c   skim milk
4   boneless, skinless, each
1 Tbsp olive oil

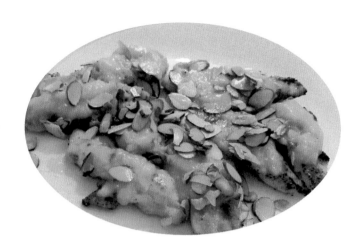

chicken breasts, 4 ounces

Heat oven to 400 F. Lightly coat a baking sheet with cooking spray. In a medium bowl, combine the ground almonds, flour, thyme, onion powder, garlic powder, salt and pepper. Pour the milk in a separate medium-sized bowl. Coat each chicken breast in the almond mixture, then into the milk, and back into the almond mixture, and place on the baking sheet.

Preheat a nonstick sauté pan on medium high heat, and add the olive oil to the pan. Once the pan is hot, place the chicken breasts in the pan and reduce heat to medium. Sear the chicken breasts on one side until they are golden brown, then sear on the other side for 1 minute. Place chicken back on the greased baking sheet and bake in the oven for about 10 minutes or until the internal temperature reaches 165 F.

EZ-PZ Pizza

Purchased whole-wheat pizza shell
Bottled pizza sauce
Sliced black olives
Shredded mozzarella cheese (or cheese substitute)

Spray pizza pan with olive oil spray. Place shell on pan and spray it as well. Spread pizza sauce on top. Top with black

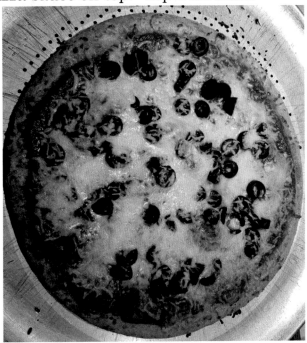

olives. Spread cheese on top.
Bake in a 450 F for 10 minutes

Noodles Romanoff

1 c cottage cheese
1 c sour cream
1 tsp soy sauce
½ tsp salt
3 c hot cooked noodles
(whole wheat is best)

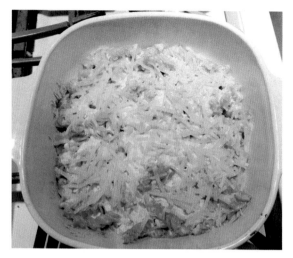

Mix all ingredients. Put in greased baking dish and top with grated cheese.
Bake at 350 degrees for 40 min.

Easy Cheese Fondue

Melt in skillet:
3 Tbsp butter
Add 3 c whole-wheat bread cubes
Put in 1 qt. greased baking disk alternating with 1 c shredded cheese.

Mix and pour over:
1 egg beaten

1 c 1 % milk
½ tsp. salt
1/8 tsp. dry mustard
Set in pan of water and bake at
350 degrees for 40 min.

Easy cheese soufflé

3 Tbsp	butter
1/4 c	grated Parmesan cheese
3 Tbsp	whole wheat flour
1 c	1% milk
1 c	shredded cheddar cheese
½ tsp	salt
1 Tbsp	mustard
3 eggs	separated
1/4 tsp	cream of tartar

Place oven rack in middle position and heat oven to 350.
Grease the bottom and sides of a meat loaf pan (about 8 ½ x 4 ½)
Sprinkle Parmesan in pan to coat.
Melt butter in microwave (about 30 seconds). Put in small
saucepan and stir in flour with a wire whisk. Cook until golden.
Slowly whisk in milk until thickened and smooth. Transfer to
large bowl. Add cheese, salt and mustard, then whisk in egg
yolks.
In a separate bowl, beat egg whites with cream of tartar with an
electric mixer until it forms stiff peaks.

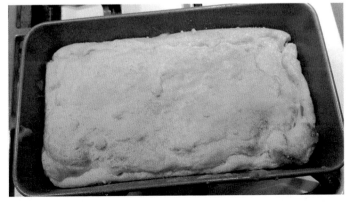

Fold whipped eggs whites slowly into yolk mixture until there are few white streaks. Pour into the prepared pan and sprinkle with the Parmesan.

Bake until nicely browned, about 30 minutes. Serves 4.

Tofu curry with mustard greens

14-16 oz.	extra-firm tofu, cut
3 Tbsp plus 2 tsp extra-virgin olive oil	
¾ tsp	fine sea salt
¼ tsp	mustard seeds
1 c	finely diced onion
2 cloves	garlic, minced
1 Tbsp	minced fresh ginger
1 ½ tsp	ground turmeric
½ tsp.	cumin seeds, toasted and ground
½ tsp.	black sesame
½ tsp.	chili powder
¼ tsp.	freshly ground black pepper
¼ tsp.	garlic powder
¼ tsp.	ground ginger
1 (14 oz.)	can chopped tomatoes with juice
1 heaping	Tbsp chunky peanut butter
1	jalapeno chili, seeds and minced
3 c	vegetable stock
12 oz	mustard greens, stems removed, but into bite-size pieces
2 Tbsp	chopped cilantro
1 c	pineapple chunks

Preheat oven to 450 degrees. Line a rimmed baking sheet with parchment paper.

Put the tofu in a bowl, drizzle with 2 tsp. of the oil, and sprinkle with ¼ tsp. of the salt. Gently toss the tofu with clean hands until evenly coated. Transfer to the lined baking sheet, spreading the tofu in a single layer. Bake, turning once after 15 minutes, for 30 minutes until firm.

Meanwhile, warm the remaining 3 Tbsp oil in a large sauté pan over medium heat. Add the mustard seeds and cook, shaking the pan occasionally, until they pop, 2 to 3 minutes. Add the onion and the remaining ½ tsp. salt and sauté until soft for 5 to 7 minutes. Add the garlic, fresh ginger, turmeric, cumin, cardamom, chili powder, black pepper, garlic powder, and ground ginger and sauté until fragrant, about 2 minutes. Add the tomatoes, peanut butter, and jalapeno and stir until well combined. Stir in the stock, mustard, greens, and bay leaves and bring to a simmer. Decrease the heat to medium-low, partially cover, and simmer, stirring occasionally, for 20 minutes.

Gently stir in the tofu and cook for 10 minutes. Remove the bay leaves. Taste and season with more salt and black pepper if desired. Serve garnished with the cilantro.
-Barbara Freeman

Sesame Noodles

8 oz package Udon noodles
3 cloves garlic minced
6 Tbsp dark sesame oil
8 oz scallions
8 oz snap peas
6 Tbsp soy sauce

Bring a pot of lightly salted water to boil. Add Udon, cooking according to instructions. In a wok or frying pan, sauté chopped scallions with garlic in dark sesame oil about 8 min. Add snap peas and sauté another 5-8 min, maintaining crispness.

Add cooked noodles and soy sauce, add more according to taste.
-Linda Mackos

Side dishes

Orange Rice

1 cup brown rice
2 cups liquid (water or orange juice)
2 tbsp. zest of an orange
½ cup yellow raisins

Lightly toast grain with or without oil, stirring, so that there are no clumps.

Add all other ingredients and cook for 30 – 40 minutes until liquid is absorbed.

Brown Rice Casserole
(Makes two casseroles. Freezes well.)

1½ cups brown rice
6 medium peppers (red and/or green)
1 large head cauliflower
2 large broccolis
1 lb. mushrooms
1 lb. Swiss cheese (you may use ½ lb. Swiss and ½ lb. cheddar)
        or 1 lb. of tofu cut into small pieces

Sauté peppers (in about 6 pieces) in olive oil slowly covered for about 20 min. Remove cover and sauté 10 min. more. Remove peppers to bowl and add salt and garlic powder to taste. Sauté mushrooms in same pan slowly covered for 10 min. Remove cover and sauté 10 min. more. Add oil if necessary. Sauté cauliflower on medium in same pan covered for 20 minutes. Cut florets off head and divide. Add a ¼ cup water. Add more water as needed. Remove cauliflower to bowl and sprinkle with Tamari lightly. Sauté broccoli florets in same pan covered for 20 minutes. Add more water as needed. Remove broccoli to bowl and sprinkle with Tamari lightly.

Sauté small pieces of the tofu in same pan if you are substituting this for cheese. Remove tofu to bowl and sprinkle with Tamari lightly. Cook brown rice with broth from pan and ½ vegetable broth and ½ water for 31/4 cups liquid. Use drippings in pepper bowl to coat casserole bottom lightly. (Use two casseroles.) Add thin layer of brown rice. Then layer with peppers, mushrooms, cauliflower and broccoli. Sprinkle with layer of shredded cheese or tofu sautéed in remaining oil after the broccoli. Combine any remaining liquid in bowl add 4 tablespoons tamari and sprinkle over both casseroles.

Bake at 350 degrees about 30 - 45 minutes until it bubbles slightly.

-Deb Hagenbuch

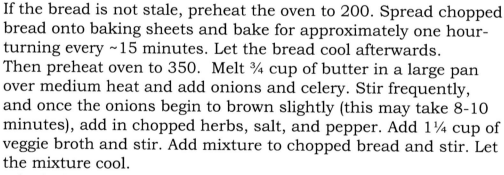

Rachel's Vegetarian- But Doesn't Taste Vegetarian- Stuffing

1½ sticks of butter
1 lb of stale bread (we usually use potato)- chopped into 1"x1" pieces
1 large chopped yellow onion
1½ cups of chopped celery
2 large eggs
Seasonings: fresh parsley, sage, rosemary and thyme (all chopped- approximately 2 tablespoons of each)
Salt and pepper to taste (use less salt if baking with salted butter)
2½ cups low-sodium vegetable broth
Cooking spray

If the bread is not stale, preheat the oven to 200. Spread chopped bread onto baking sheets and bake for approximately one hour- turning every ~15 minutes. Let the bread cool afterwards.
Then preheat oven to 350. Melt ¾ cup of butter in a large pan over medium heat and add onions and celery. Stir frequently, and once the onions begin to brown slightly (this may take 8-10 minutes), add in chopped herbs, salt, and pepper. Add 1¼ cup of veggie broth and stir. Add mixture to chopped bread and stir. Let the mixture cool.
Whisk the remaining 1¼ cup of broth and 2 eggs in a bowl. Add to the cooled bread mixture and stir gently until everything is combined. Spray a 13"x9" dish generously with cooking spray. Add the bread mixture to the dish.Cook the stuffing, covered with foil, for approximately 40 minutes. Uncover the stuffing, and continue to cook for another 40-45 minutes, or until the top is brown and crispy.
Note, if making in advance, you can cook the stuffing for 40 minutes and then put in the refrigerator. Take it out and bake it uncovered. If cooking from chilled, add another 10 minutes.
　　　　　　　-Rachel Franceschino

Vegetables

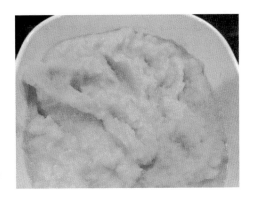

Baked squash

Cut butternut squash in half and scoop out seeds. Bake in 350 degree oven for one hour. Remove skin and mash with margarine and a small amount of brown sugar. Heat for ten more minutes.

Carrots with butter and dried parsley

Wash carrots and cut into small pieces. Dot with butter and dried parsley. Bake in 350 F oven for 45 minutes or until tender.

Food

Butternut Squash with Whole Wheat, Wild Rice, & Onion Stuffing

4 medium-small butternut squashes (about 1 pound each)
¾ cup raw wild rice, rinsed
1½ Tbsp olive oil
1 large red onion
2 to 3 cloves garlic, minced
2½ cups firmly packed torn whole wheat bread
        (use gluten-free bread if you'd like)
1 Tbsp sesame seeds
A few sliced fresh sage leaves (or leave whole if small), optional
½ tsp. dried thyme
1 Tbsp salt-free mixed season blend (such as Frontier or Mrs. Dash), or to taste
½ c vegetable broth
Juice of 1 small orange (about ¼ cup; or omit and just use more vegetable broth)
Salt and freshly ground pepper to taste.

Preheat the oven to 375 degrees F.
Wrap the whole squashes in foil. Place on a rack in the center of the oven. Bake for 40 to 45 minutes, or until you can pierce through the narrow part with a knife, with a little resistance. You can do this step ahead of time. Let the squashes cool somewhat, then cut in half lengthwise, and scoop out the seeds and their surrounding fibers.

Meanwhile, bring 2 cups of water to a boil in a saucepan. Stir in the wild rice, reduce to a simmer, then cover and cook until the water is absorbed, about 40 minutes. Heat the oil in a skillet. Add the onion and garlic and sauté until golden. In a mixing bowl, combine the cooked wild rice with the sautéed onion and the remaining ingredients (whole wheat bread sprinkled with salt and pepper).

Scoop out the squash pulp, leaving firm shells about ½ inch thick.

Page 131

Chop or dice the pulp and stir it into the wild rice mixture. Stuff the squashes, place in foil-lined baking dishes, and cover. Place the squashes in a preheated 350 Degree F. oven. Bake for 15 to 20 minutes, or just until well heated through.

Cauliflower au Gratin

Cook cauliflower in water with rice vinegar until tender but still crisp. Spread on a baking pan. Top with cubed cheddar cheese. Add whole wheat raisin bread (or plain whole wheat bread) which has been sautéed in butter or oil. Bake at 350 degrees for 15 minutes. Garnish with fresh parsley if desired.

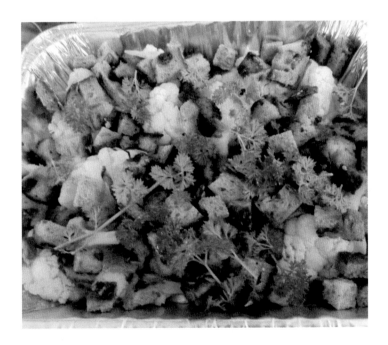

Breads

Banana muffins

3   very ripe bananas mashed
½ c. vanilla almond milk (or 1% milk + 1 tsp. Vanilla)
1 c.   sugar
2 c.   whole wheat or oat flour
1 tsp. baking soda
½ tsp. cinnamon
¼ tsp salt

Preheat oven to 350 degrees.
In a large bowl, whisk together flour, sugar, baking soda, salt and cinnamon. In a medium bowl, mash your bananas with a fork, then whisk in the milk and vanilla (if using). Fold the dry into the wet till fully incorporated using a fork.
Line muffin pans with paper liners. Scoop batter (about 2 Tbsp per cup). Bake for 22 - 26 minutes until golden brown and toothpick inserted in center comes out clean. Top with a dollop of peanut butter and banana slices.

Gluten-free Carrot Raisin Muffins

2 c   almond flour
¼ c   chopped walnuts
¼ c   raisins
½ tsp   cinnamon
½ tsp   baking soda
1/8 tsp sea salt
3   eggs or substitute applesauce, bananas or pumpkin
1 c   shredded carrots
¼ c   maple syrup
2 Tbsp olive oil
1 tsp   apple cider vinegar

Preheat oven to 325 degrees. Grease or line muffin tin.
Combine dry ingredients in large bowl. Combine wet ingredients
in medium bowl. Stir these into dry ingredients. Bake for 20-25
minutes.

Pumpkin muffins

8 oz.	silken tofu
8 oz.	canned pureed pumpkin
¾ c	brown sugar
½ c	applesauce
½ c	apple juice
2 c	whole wheat flour
2 tsp	baking soda
1 tsp	baking powder
1 tsp	pumpkin pie spice
¼ tsp	cinnamon
1 tsp	vanilla extract
½ c	raisins (optional)

Preheat oven to 350 degrees.
Puree tofu and pumpkin in a blender. Add sugar, applesauce
and apple juice. Blend until smooth. In a separate bowl,
combine dry ingredients. Add pumpkin mixture to dry
ingredients and mix until combined. Add raisins. Fill greased
muffin pan and bake for 10 - 12 minutes.

Salads

Cranberry Pecan Wild Rice Salad

1   shallot, chopped
1 tsp garlic salt
1 tsp. dried rosemary
1 c   wild rice, rinsed and drained
3 c   vegetable broth
2 c   mandarin orange juice
½ c   dried cranberries
2 Tbsp pure maple syrup
1 Tbsp Dijon mustard
1 Tbsp Tamari (optional) or 1 tsp. salt
½ c.   chopped pecans

Sauté onion and garlic in 1/4 c. vegetable broth over medium heat, about six minutes. Add rosemary by crushing it between your fingers as you sprinkle it in. Add the wild rice, remaining vegetable broth, mandarin juice and dried cranberries. Bring to a boil, cover, reduce heat and simmer for 45 -50 minutes until the rice is cooked through, chewy but not hard. If there is any liquid remaining, cook uncovered for another 5 minutes. Remove from heat, stir in maple syrup, Dijon and tamari until incorporated. Add nuts and stir to combine. May be served warm or at room temperature.

Waldorf salad

Combine cubed apples (organic preferred) with sliced celery, raisins (or dates) and cut-up pecans. Stir in low-fat mayonnaise with a small amount of whipped cream. Sprinkle with cinnamon.

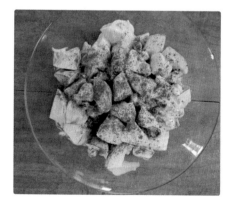

Tossed salad

Wash lettuce and tomatoes. Top organic romaine lettuce and organic cherry tomatoes with olives and shredded cheese.

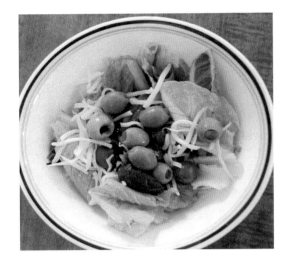

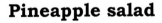

Pear salad

Top canned pears which have been drained with dates, dried cranberries and coconut.

Pineapple salad

Combine drained canned pineapple chunks with coconut and dates.

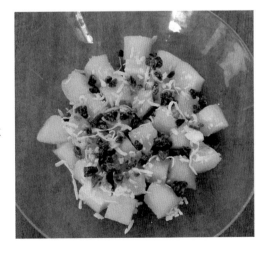

Peach salad

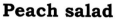
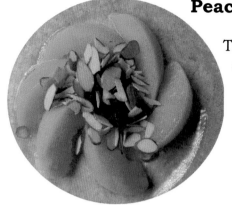

Top canned peaches with sliced almonds and dates.

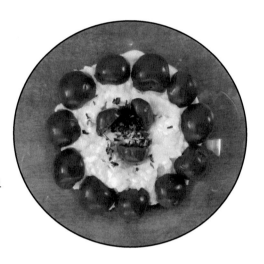

Tomato salad

Combine cherry tomatoes with low-fat cottage cheese.

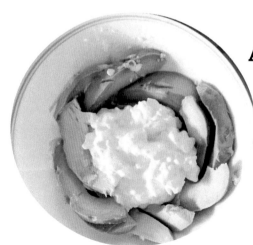

Avocado salad

Arrange avocado slices around low-fat cottage cheese.

Carrot salad

Shred carrots. Combine with shredded coconut and raisins. Combine mayonnaise and whipped cream. Mix with carrot mixture.

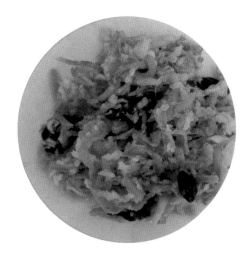

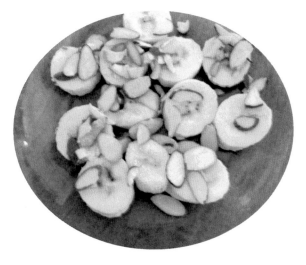

Cole slaw

Shred cabbage and carrots. Mix mayonnaise with small amount of mustard and combine with cabbage. Top with parsley, if desired.

Bananas with sliced almonds

Slice bananas. Sprinkle with Fruit Fresh or a little orange juice to prevent browning. Top with sliced almonds.

Snacks

Warm Chipotle Black Bean Dip
10-12 servings
Prep time: 30 mins
Cook time: 15 mins

2 Tbsp olive oil
1 large yellow onion, diced
3 cloves garlic, minced
1 Tbsp chili powder
2 cans black beans (31 oz total), drained and rinsed, divided
1 can chipotle chilies in adobo sauce
¾ cup water
3 tbsp apple cider vinegar
1 (14.5 oz) can diced tomatoes, drained
1½ cups frozen corn, thawed
6 oz shredded sharp Cheddar cheese, divided
6 oz shredded sharp Monterey Jack cheese, divided
¾ cup chopped fresh cilantro
Salt and pepper, to taste

Preheat oven to 425 degrees. Spray a 1½ quart baking dish with non-stick cooking spray and place on a foil-lined baking sheet and set aside.

Chop 2 chipotle chilies, set aside 3 tbsp adobo sauce from can. Heat oil in a large skillet over medium high heat. Reduce to medium and add onion and salt, cooking about 4 to 6 minutes until onion is softened and translucent. Add garlic and chili powder, stir for 1 minute. Add chopped chilies, adobo sauce, water, and half the black beans. Bring to a boil and cook until the liquid reduces by half, about 2 to 3 minutes.

Transfer bean mixture to a blender or food processor, add vinegar and process until completely smooth. Allow mixture to cool for 5 minutes then transfer to a large bowl. Stir in remaining beans, tomatoes, corn, half of both cheeses, and ½ cup of cilantro. Season with salt and pepper to taste.

Transfer mixture to baking dish and cover with remaining cheese. Bake until the cheese is melted and slightly browned around edges, about 15 minutes. Garnish with remaining cilantro and serve warm with tortilla chips.
   -*Sarah Koontz*

Endurance crackers

½ c.   chia seeds
½ c.   sunflower seeds
½ c.   pumpkin seeds (or Pepita seeds)
½ c.   sesame seeds
1 c.   water
1   garlic clove, finely grated
1 tsp grated sweet onion
¼ tsp kosher salt
       Herb Amare and kelp granules (optional)

Preheat oven to 325 degrees and line a large baking sheet with parchment paper.

In a large bowl, mix the seeds together. In a small bowl, mix the water, grated garlic and grated onion. Whisk well. Pour the water mixture onto the seeds and stir until thick and combined. Season with salt, and optional Herb Amare and kelp granules, to taste. Add spices or fresh herbs if you wish. Spread the mixture onto the prepared baking sheet with the back of a spoon until it is less than ¼ inch thick. Do not worry if a part becomes too thin, you can just patch them up.

Bake for 30 minutes. Remove from oven, slice into crackers, carefully flip onto the other side with a spatula. Bake for another 30 minutes, watching closely after about 25 minutes. The bottoms will be lightly golden in color. Allow to cool completely on the pan. Store in a container.
   -Angela Liddon

Vegan Energy Bar

½ c	whole-wheat flour
2/3 c	oatmeal
1 c.	Grape Nuts cereal
¾ c	raisins
1 c	shredded coconut
1/3 c	unsalted almonds, chopped
1/3 c	unsalted cashews, chopped
1	cinnamon stick, ground or 2 tsp ground
2 Tbsp	flax seed
¼ c	warm water
1½ c	cooked kidney beans (or 1 15 oz. can)
15	pitted dates, chopped
1 tsp	vanilla extract
2 Tbsp	honey
1 Tbsp	canola oil
½ c	applesauce

Preheat oven to 350 degrees.
Unless canned, kidney beans should be soaked overnight, then simmered for about one hour or until soft. If canned, rinse well. Chop the beans roughly either by hand or by a food processor just until tiny pieces. Grind the flax seed and mix it with the water, set aside to thicken. Combine the dry ingredients and mix well. Add the wet ingredients and mix until uniformly combined. Press into a greased 9 x 13″ pan or casserole dish. Bake for a total of 20 - 25 minutes, rotating half way through. Cool completely then cut into 24 bars.

Store unwrapped for harder bars, put in an airtight container for softer bars. Toast cut bars in a toaster oven for a crispy outside. If keeping longer than one week, wrap and freeze.

Nutrition facts for one bar: 157 kcal., 38.3 kcal. fat, sat. fat 1.25%, protein 4.6 %, sodium 66 %, sugar 13.9 %, fiber 7.4%.

-Angela Liddon

Thai Peanut Popcorn

½ c	popcorn kernels
2 Tbsp	maple syrup
1 Tbsp	sugar
2 Tbsp	peanut butter
1 to 2 tsp	hot sauce to taste
¼ tsp	garlic powder
½ c	roasted peanuts

Pop popcorn in a microwave popper or a paper lunch bag with the top folded over until popping slows to a few seconds. Pour into a bowl. In a small saucepan bring the honey and sugar to a simmer and cook for two minutes. Remove from heat, add peanut butter, hot sauce and garlic powder. Add peanuts and stir well. Cool for 10 -15 minutes.

Peanut butter crunch cups

1½ c	puffed quinoa
¼ c + 2 Tbsp	peanut butter
2 Tbsp	canola oil
1½ Tbsp	maple syrup
1 tsp	vanilla extract

Put paper liners in muffin cups (16 - 18).

In medium bowl add puffed quinoa. Combine peanut butter, oil, maple syrup and vanilla in medium saucepan. Heat over low heat, whisk for 4 -5 minutes or until completely melted and smooth. Pour over quinoa and stir to coat. Drop heaping tablespoons of the mixture into the muffin cups. Pop into the freezer for one hour. Once set, transfer to the refrigerator.

-Ashley Melillo

Roasted Chickpeas
Makes about 1 cup

1 can	chickpeas
1 tsp	olive oil
¼ tsp	salt
½ tsp	garlic powder
½ tsp	dried basil
1 tsp	nutritional yeast (or Parmesan cheese)
¼ tsp	red pepper flakes

Drain and rinse the chickpeas, then pat them dry. In a small mixing bowl, combine the chickpeas, oil, and seasonings. Mix until everything is evenly coated. Pour the chickpeas onto a baking pan covered in aluminum foil and shake gently until the chickpeas are in one layer.

Roast at 450 degrees for 10-15 minutes, toss, and roast for another 10-15 minutes until golden and beginning to brown. Turn off the oven, crack it open, and let the chickpeas cool for another 20 minutes (this will keep them even crispier!). Serve at room temperature as a snack or toss into a salad.

-Tammy Tenerowitz

Healthier Chex mix

Melt 3 tbsp butter in the microwave. Mix in 2 tbsp soy sauce.
Sprinkle on 1 tbsp of onion salt. Mix together 2 c whole wheat
Chex cereal, 2 c rice Chex, 2 c corn Chex and 1 c peanuts. Pour
liquid over and mix. Put into 350 Degree oven for one hour,
taking out to stir every 15 minutes. Spray with olive oil and
serve.

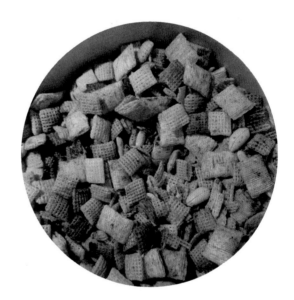

Healthy popcorn

Airpop popcorn kernels in the
microwave. Spray with olive oil
and sprinkle with salt to taste.

Food

Chapter thirteen
Not in my back yard

Waste not, want not

We tend to forget how lucky we are. If you go camping in a tent, you will appreciate running water and flush toilets when you get back home. (I can vouch for that.) Not everyone in the world has these conveniences. We take a lot of things for granted, like being warm in the winter and cool in the summer.

Keeping it cold

Refrigeration is another thing we take for granted. If your power goes out because of a storm, your refrigerator may be the first concern. Keeping food cold is important in order to prevent spoilage, and unsafe food. I am old enough to remember (barely) an ice box which relied on someone who delivered a block of ice to the "ice box" in your kitchen. The ice was cut from lakes in the winter and stored in straw or underground in the warmer months. There is a place near my home where they celebrate an ice harvest every winter, in remembrance of days gone by.

Unfortunately, refrigeration is something that contributes greatly to global climate change. The old types of refrigerants, CFCs and HCFCs (types of chlorofluorocarbons) were depleting the ozone layer thus allowing more ultraviolet rays to reach the earth. They were found in refrigerators, air conditioning units, aerosol cans and dry-cleaning agents. They have been phased out, but some are still around. Fortunately, there was an agreement in 2016 by 170 countries to phase out these chemicals. (1) That is the good news.

Food

According to the book, *Drawdown: the most Comprehensive Plan ever Proposed to Reverse Global Warming,* the bad news is that the replacement, HFCs (hydro fluorocarbons) warm the atmosphere in an amount thousands of times greater than carbon dioxide does. (2) The price of cooling inside is warming outside. Put your hand near the output of your refrigerator or air conditioner and you will get the idea.

Thus, open your refrigerator door as little as possible - good advice even without a power outage. Line up the things to put in your refrigerator and put them in all at once. Complain to your supermarket about their open refrigerator units. If possible, don't buy large freezers. They do have a large impact on your electric bill.

Use it up - leftovers become new dishes

It is possible to plan one meal with enough leftovers to make a new dish. This puts your creative genes to good use. I know from experience that the results can be mixed, and not always tasty. However, it is a good way to save time while using up what might go in the garbage (or compost pot). An example would be to bake a chicken one day with a side of rice. Then cut the chicken up for a chicken-rice casserole or chicken rice soup the next. Perhaps your turkey can become layered with stuffing, vegetables and gravy.

Store leftovers on one or two shelves in your refrigerator where you will notice them, and try to bring things in the back forward. The point is to use up as much as possible.

Compost

Leftovers that you can't find new uses for can become compost in the backyard. Vegetable peelings are great for composting. If you have a space away from the house, start a compost pile for later use in the garden. A pot with a secure lid can be used to store the leftovers on the way to the compost pile.

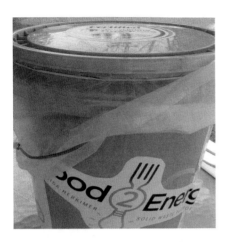

This is my compost pot. It is collected every two weeks, and becomes energy for the local waste treatment plant. (3)

Locally we have a small business that provides a compost pot for food scraps and collects the scraps every two weeks. These provide fuel for a new anaerobic incinerator at our county waste-management center.(3) My daughter tells me that when they stayed in London in an apartment, they were supplied with a compost pot that was put out with the garbage for collection. When we travel, we notice some of the airports have separate containers for waste, recycling and compost.

Food Banks

Some restaurants, school and college food services have agreements with community food banks to take the leftover food. College students may act as volunteers to deliver the food in a timely manner. Health requirements are a concern and there are limitations here. Every community has people in need and thus this provides a humanitarian as well as an environmental purpose.

Paper is for walls

Limit your use of paper as much as possible. Wallpaper looks pretty on your walls and lasts a long time, but wet, soggy paper does not look good in the landfills. If you ever visited a paper plant, you don't forget the awful, chemical smell. most paper mills uses many caustic chemicals which become pollutants. The process also requires fossil-fuel-driven boilers. (4) To obtain the wood that becomes paper requires cutting down many trees. As mentioned before, trees are a great engine for taking carbon dioxide out of the air, thus helping to counteract climate change.

Food

Instead of paper napkins, use wash cloths. They are absorbent and easy to toss in the washing machine. Each member of the family can have a different color. Use small cloths or sponges for washing dishes and cleaning. Instead of paper towels, use a cloth or sponge. Sponges can be put in the microwave for two minutes to sanitize them. (Do that every day or two.)

Recycling

In our small community, the village highway department crew picks up large items we put at the curb on a certain day. In many instances, these are picked up early by someone who finds that *one person's junk is another person's treasure.* An even better plan is to take these to an organization such as Goodwill, the Salvation Army, a veterans' organization or Habitat for Humanity. If you have a large item, most organizations will send a truck to pick it up. You will even get a receipt so that you can get a tax deduction.

Metal and copper are much in demand. Where we live, people will come by and pick up any metal and take it to a recycling business in exchange for cash. Most disappears in a very short time.

We are lucky to have an excellent recycling center in our area. It is called "single stream" which means that everything except food waste and

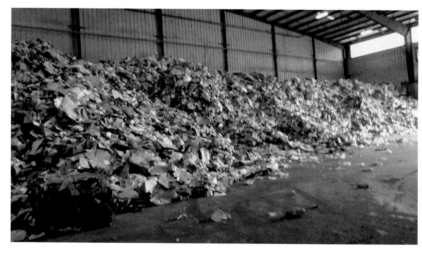

Part of one day's garbage at the recycling cneter

some plastics can be combined in one bin for pickup. Much of the waste stream is sorted by large machines and sold for various reuses. An example is plastic bottles, which can be turned into decking and components of roads. Food waste is turned into compost. Newspapers become reused paper. Look for recycled paper when you buy paper products at the store such as toilet paper and paper towels. Take a tour of your recycling center as we did, and you will be amazed at what they can do.

Plastics were the future

Unfortunately recycling centers are currently having a problem because China is now refusing recycled materials from the U.S. China was previously a substantial importer of recycled

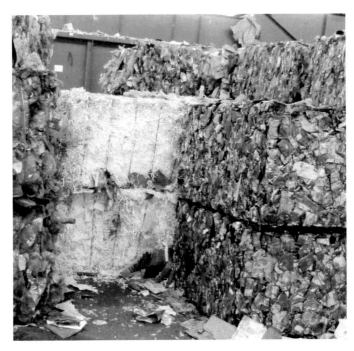

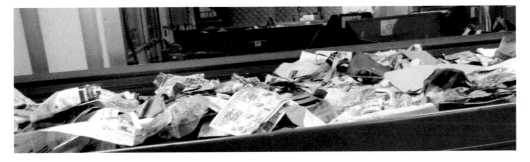

This stream of waste is separated into medal, paper and garbage at our recycling center. It still requires people along the line to take out plastic bags which get caught in the equipment, thus stopping the line.

materials, turning it into the plastic products we buy. However, the Chinese found too much contaminated material in the recycling from the U.S. People have not been cleaning the cans and bottles they put in the recycling containers. We used to have a business that reused recycled Styrofoam for packing materials. However, this was spoiled when meat trays and other unclean materials were found mixed in with the clean Styrofoam.

In New York State, single-use plastic bags have been eliminated. In two years, Styrofoam products may also be outlawed.

New companies are joining the recycling bandwagon. One in Trenton, New Jersey called Terra Cycle turns waste into usable products. Some companies such as Subaru autos, Brita filters and Colgate will even provide padded envelope with a shipping label to send to this recycling company. These are free. Larger boxes may be purchased by a business or organization. (5) Such things as a used toothbrush, a water filter, a chip bag, disposable cups and other items bound for the waste stream, can be cleaned and shredded to become a park bench or supplies for schools. Zero

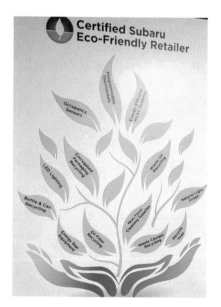

This recycling container was found at my local Subaru dealer.

This poster highlights the various ways in which this dealer is pursuing a environmentally-friendly path.

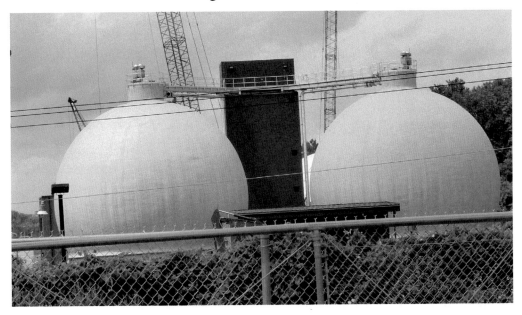

These are the anaerobic digesters at our recycling center which produce all the fuel needed to run the entire facility.

Waste Boxes can be found at various Subaru dealerships. (6)(

Not in my back yard

Buying for the long term is also a smart strategy, not only for saving money, but for reducing the amount that contributes to our landfill problem. No one seems to want a landfill in their backyard. Many landfills contribute methane to the atmosphere, a potent greenhouse gas. Newer anaerobic digesters are turning refuse into fuel.

Also, as we are transitioning to a digital world, hopefully there will be less to recycle. Remember that your old computers and printers can also be recycled at your local recycling center. There are companies that pick these up and take them apart to reclaim the precious elements that they contain.

Food

Hints:

Be sure to put only clean materials in your recycling container.
Use cloth reusable bags for purchases.
Buy things that last as LONG as possible.

Chapter fourteen
Food for the future

New advances are being made in the production, transportation and types of food.

Robots, drones and sensors - oh my

Just like Dorothy in her search for the Wizard of Oz, we are searching for a technology to make food more available, more reasonably priced, and even better for the environment.

Increasingly we are being taken over by technology in many areas. Robots are one example. Sometimes this is bad - meaning

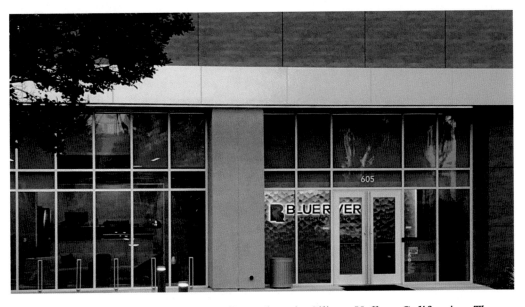

This is the entrance to the Blue River plant in Silicon Valley. California. They manufacture special robots that target weeds called the Lettuce Bot. Photo by Kevin Reardon.

the loss of jobs. However, sometimes this is good - replacing back-breaking labor by humans with special robots.

One example is the new See and Spray. Developed by a small start-up company in the Silicon Valley of California called Blue River, it has been bought by John Deere, that giant company that is synonymous with large tractors. It was founded by Jorgé Heraud. (1)

In Chapter Three we laid out the case for no-till farming. This is still practiced on only one-fifth of farms in this country and only ten percent globally. (2) One problem is the invasive weeds such as pigweed that are nearly impossible to control. (I regretfully have some invasive weeds in my small, backyard garden which seem impossible to eradicate.)

Using lots and lots of trial and error, a special robot was developed. It looks at healthy plants and learns to distinguish them from weeds. When attached to a special tractor it can spray herbicide on only the weeds, leaving the healthy plants alone to thrive. The first experimental models decimated whole fields of crops. However, after much experimentation, the LettuceBot was perfected. It is designed to recognize healthy lettuce plants and spray only the weeds surrounding them.(3) Now they are working on developing a memory bank for cotton. Hopefully other plants will follow. (I would love that in my home garden.)

The result is much lower production costs because of reduced use of herbicides. Also, the vegetable is much safer for the consumer.

Growing up and not getting dirty

If there is not enough land to grow the food you need, the answer may be vertical farming. Especially in countries such as China and Japan there is a need to feed a growing population with insufficient good-quality soil. The demand for organic food is expanding in these countries as well as in the U.S.

Saving transportation costs by growing food closer to urban areas saves not only money, but limits greenhouse-gas emissions. Surprisingly this is happening in the U.S. *One of the largest vertical-farming companies in the world is unassumingly headquartered in an old laser-tag building in ... Newark, New Jersey.* (4) This company is named AeroFarms because it grows plants in air inside a windowless building.

These operations require the extensive use of artificial light, though LEDs are now being used. The combination of high-intensity blue-and red-spectrum light mimics the light of the sun. This is similar to my kitchen garden mentioned in Chapter nine, though on a giant scale.

The beds are made of a type of fabric, rather than soil. The developer, Ed Harwood, originally found this fleece-type fabric in Jo-Ann's (one of my favorite stores) in Ithaca, New York. He was a professor and administrator at Cornell University. (5) (He also developed an ankle-bracelet for cows that used their movement to determine if they were fertile. He was a very creative inventor.)

He began in a rented basement workspace near Ithaca. He started with seeds for arugula spread on the fabric placed in long boxes. Mixing water with a homemade nutrient mixture, he sprayed the plants, and had a harvest in a mere two weeks. He put this plan on a website and forgot about it, until some investors saw the potential. The result is the Newark factory.

The factory is high-tech using oxygen to speed growth. It also requires cameras and precision use of soil sensors and data networks to be effective.

This is an application of food production that will probably grow, but according to Paul Hawken *will not alone reduce greenhouse gas emissions, nor will it alone feed the population.* (6)

Food

Greenhouses grow large

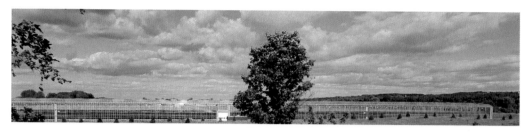

Green Enpire Farms in upstate New York is a new giant greenhouse. By using sustainable methods, they are growing produce indoors under controlled conditions.

Located in central New York is a commercial greenhouse built in 2020. Owned by a Canadian company, it is an expanded idea of an old concept. Greenhouses have long been used to grow vegetables and flowers on a small scale. However, Green Empire Farms rests on a huge plot - 32 acres of land. (7)

The concept is to grow produce such as strawberries and tomatoes when the weather outside is "frightful." In other words, summer produce can be grown all year round. The plants are waist-high for easy maintenance and picking. The glass is especially slanted in a diamond shape to direct more of the suns' rays inside, especially since this is an area known for cloudy days.

Part of the plan is the use of natural methods to fight pests. Lady bugs are encouraged because they eat aphids. Bee hives are an important part for pollination, and they are protected from external pesticides.

Unfortunately, in 2020 this farm was better known for the growth of Covid-19 in May. The need for seasonal workers who lived closely in neighboring hotels exacerbated the spread of the virus. The managers of the facility are quickly building living facilities for the workers and instituting measures to provide separation when the workers are on-the-job.

In this year of the great pandemic, a similar situation has occurred in meat-packing plants where working conditions have necessitated close working conditions. As Andrew Cuomo, Governor of New York, stated, *"it is not the meat or the produce causing the problem, it is the proximity of the workers."* (8)

Perhaps when the pandemic is not the top news story, the idea of these modern greenhouses may prove to be the future of produce production. The use of sustainable methods is to be commended, as long as the workers are protected and compensated reasonably well.

New Superfoods

Developing a taste for beetles and other bugs may not be an appetizing alternative for the McDonalds generation. However, they have been used in some countries for generations, and are surprisingly high in protein.

Other foods that seem more palatable and may increase in usage in the near future are grains such as quinoa. It uses less water, survives in salty soil, and is high in protein. (9) It is being bred to be less bitter and produce higher yields.

Moringa is another grain that has not as yet become popular. Researchers funded by the Bill and Melinda Gates Foundation are experimenting with gene-editing techniques to make possible higher-volume harvests. Supposedly this would help subsistence farmers in India and other third-world countries. (10)

However, an organization called GRAIN developed to help these small farmers argues that most of the Gates Foundation money is being directed to scientists in the U.S. in a top-down approach. GRAIN suggests that small farmers have experience and expertise in growing crops and are not being consulted. Powerful transnational corporations are taking more land, incorporating GMOs and increased use of fertilizer. (11)

Food

What's the new beef?

Artificial meat is growing in popularity. It is not meat at all. Impossible Foods is one of the leaders in this technology. In May 2019 it was valued at $2 billion on the stock market. Quite a feat for a company that started in 2011. The most well-known product is the Impossible Burger which was launched in July 2016. (12)

A professor at Stanford, Patrick Brown, became concerned about the huge role that animal farming has on the environment. (Hopefully you remember that this was discussed in Chapter Five.) He founded a company, Impossible Foods, to develop a substitute for the ever-popular burger (a staple of so many diets and fast-food chains). It claims to have 30% less sodium and 40% less saturated fat, no gluten, and as much protein as ground beef. (13)

The scientists first studied the elements of the beef burger that give it the signature taste. A major factor is heme, the substance that makes blood red (which causes me to faint) and carries oxygen through living organisms. It is also found in plant sources such as wheat, potato and a small amount of coconut fat. When it was tested to be GRS (Generally Recognized as Safe) in 2014, it hit the market with a vengeance.

This new meat is even being incorporated in the menus of some of the large fast-food chains such as White Castle and Burger King. Next is pizza with sausage made from plants possibly coming to your local Little Caesars.

Another company, Memphis Meats, based in Berkeley, California, was founded by Uma Valeti, a cardiologist, and Nicholas Genovese, a stem cell biologist. (14) They develop meat from the cells of animals, thereby eliminating the messy slaughter of living beings. These cells are grown in a laboratory instead.

In 2018 this company was purchased by Tyson Foods, a company that produces 20% of the meat consumed in the U.S. This company has also been jointly sued by *Earth and Water Watch* and *Organic Consumers Association* for deceptive advertising. The charge by these groups is that Tyson practices inhumane treatment of chickens, and dispenses toxic pollutants into waterways in the U.S. (15) In 2020 Tyson has been cited for poor working conditions resulting in more COVID-19 cases among its workers.

Beyond Meat produces another meat substitute. They produce the Beyond Burger. The ingredients listed are: water, pea protein isolate, expeller-pressed canola oil, refined coconut oil, rice protein, natural flavors, cocoa butter, mung bean protein, methylcellulose, potato starch, apple extract, salt, potassium chloride, vinegar, lemon juice concentrate, sunflower, lecithin, pomegranate fruit powder, beet juice extract (for color). It certainly takes a lot of ingredients to imitate meat. High in protein and free of gluten, this may be an alternative for some.

A third beef-patty-substitute is Sweet Earth Awesome Burger. At least the name sounds appetizing.

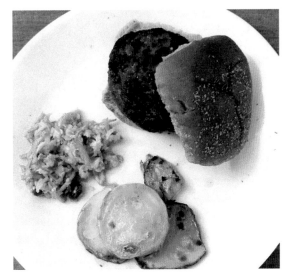

We tried one of these pseudo-meat patties for dinner. Paired with organic catsup and a whole-wheat bun, it was pretty good. However, these are highly processed foods, something we normally try to avoid. They are also expensive and high in calories. If substituted for beef, perhaps they are a good idea from an environmental standpoint.

Food

On the plus side, these burgers have no cholesterol and are high in fiber and protein. On the negative side, they are high in sodium and fat. (16)

Most of these new products were doing well in the stock market in 2019. Only time will tell what the future holds for these new meat substitutes.

Print your own dinner

Writing this on the fiftieth anniversary of the first man on the moon, I realize that a great deal of food technology was developed for space flight. Also, much of it has also been developed for the purposes of the military. The majority of this innovation has been spawned at the U.S. Army Research and Development and Engineering Center in Natick, Massachusetts. (17) The purpose is to find foods that are compact, portable, not requiring refrigeration, and yes, nutritional.

Scientists in this laboratory have developed yet another robot called a Foodini. (18) It creates an edible snack using a 3-D printer. (How scary is that?) Instead of using plastic to build a structure, it uses a soft food substance. Early models use cartridges filled with such things as pea-protein dough, avocado paste, or a chocolate-peanut butter mix. These are extruded through the cartridges to make small cubes can be quickly cooked in a microwave or chilled as needed.

Another development is to build sensors into the uniforms of soldiers to determine their health status. Perhaps in the future they will be able to determine the specific nutrient needs of the soldiers and customize the food pellets to meet those needs. (19)

Fish food

There is a laboratory in Norway specializing in development of algae called the Marine Harvest Laboratory. It is specifically located next to an oil refinery because it uses the carbon dioxide produced in the production of oil. The CO2 plus sunlight nourishes the growth of microscopic plants in glass tubes. The purpose is to develop a vegetarian diet for salmon. The algae can potentially shorten the food chain.

As noted in Chapter Six, larger fish eat smaller fish and so on down the line. The algae produce the good omega-3 fatty acids which make fish so healthy for us. As more fish farms are being developed to meet the increased need for more fish, there is demand for a more efficient way to feed them. Food pellets are being used to feed fish such as salmon instead of a diet of raw fish. The pellets also require less feed per pound of edible product.

Fish meets the protein demands of people with less cost to the environment. According to Amanda Little in her book *The Fate of Food* "*while seafood is the dominant source of protein for nearly half of humanity, relatively little of it is eaten in the industrial West.*" (20) Perhaps that will change as people become more health conscious.

Bananas and Boats

Bananas are great nutrition. They contain vitamins C and B6 plus minerals such as manganese, potassium and others. They are also a favorite food in developed countries. Americans eat 27 pounds per person every year. (21)

Some recent efforts to grow bananas in northern greenhouses are being tried. You can even buy a variety of banana plant to grow in a pot. If you have a very warm sunporch, you might give it a try.

Few of us have a banana tree in the backyard. They require a tropical environment. Bananas are also very delicate. They spoil and bruise easily, and quickly can turn black and mushy. They are picked green, wrapped carefully and kept under cool conditions. They may travel from the back of a mule to a truck to a shipping container and loaded on a huge, refrigerated ship.

The long chain of careful and mostly cool conditions is costly. It requires a great deal of energy. There is pressure to produce new refrigerated vehicles that are less expensive and have less impact on the environment.

Energy needs

The liquid Geritol has long claimed that it gives your body energy. It is composed of mostly alcohol, iron and B vitamins. As the result of lawsuits, it can only claim "to help relieve symptoms of tiredness only in persons who suffer from iron deficiency anemia", (22) We all need energy and would like to drink something to instantly feel better.

However, the world has an even bigger problem. It needs lots of energy for heat, air conditioning, refrigeration and transportation, to mention the most obvious. But there is no easy fix. The world can't down a big bottle of caffeine and instantly solve its energy problems.

Thanks to government rebates in some states, we see an increasing number of solar panels on houses and in yards, as well as commercial fields. Farmers have found that windmills help supplement their income from crops, and the wind from the ocean is also being used. In New York State, Niagara Falls is used as a source of hydro-power.

Will all of these be enough to offset fossil fuel depletion and the dangerous by-products of nuclear energy? There are scientists working on alternatives.

One fairly new energy source is hydrogen. A Department of Energy research lab in Richland, Washington is working on a way to power refrigeration trucks with hydrogen. (23)

Ships are also one of the most common methods of shipping food between countries. However, most ships use incredibly dirty fuel, even worse than the fuel used by trucks. A company in Norway christened the world's first hydrogen-powered cruise ship in 2017. (24) General Dynamics in San Diego, California developed a hydrogen-powered container ship in 2012. These are now being developed by a company in China. (25)

Hydrogen power uses a chemical reaction to produce electricity. One problem is that hydrogen is very explosive. Also, liquid hydrogen needs to be maintained at a very low temperature. The impetus is regulations by the maritime industry to reduce emissions.

According to Jeremy Rifkin in his book *The Hydrogen Economy*, hydrogen is the fuel of the future. However, that future remains to be seen. (26)

Will superfoods replace supermoms?

Will these foods catch on with the public? Are any of these new super foods better than mother's home cooking? Time will tell.

Hint

Don't be afraid to try something new.

Food

Chapter fifteen
The light at the end of the tunnel

The earth is our home. Unless we preserve the rest of life, as a sacred duty, we will be endangering ourselves by destroying the home in which we evolved, and on which we completely depend.
— Edward Osborne Wilson

When looking at the big picture of climate changes, it is easy to get discouraged. There are things that we as individuals and in close-knit groups can do to "hold back the ocean" of change.

The future lies with the young

Fortunately, young people are becoming more and more involved in issues of climate change actions. When Greta Thunberg was

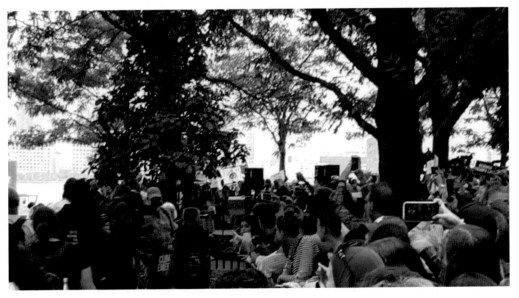

Hundreds flanked the shore in New York City to greet Greta Thunberg when she arrived on Catamarran from Europe. Photo by David Carman

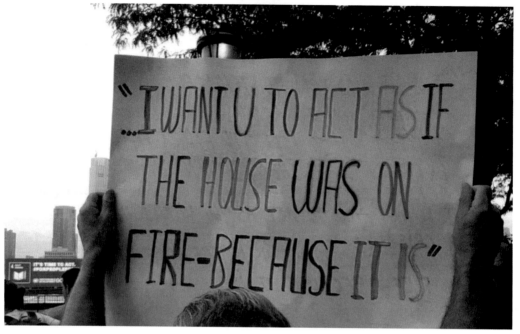

This person uses a large, hand-made sign to express her concern about the climate.

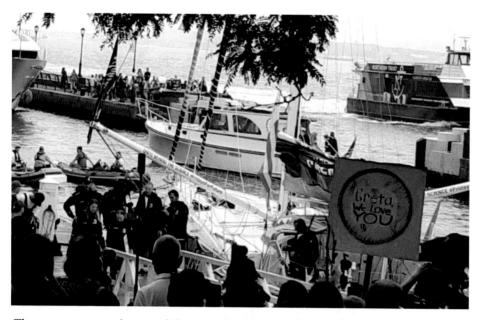

These are more photos of the people greeting Greta Thunberg when she arrived to speak at the United Nations. Photos by David Carman

named "Person of the Year" by *Time Magazine* it was a great boost to the environmental movement. The idea of a sixteen-year-old presenting to the members of the United Nations is revolutionary. (1)

Greta modeled her beliefs by taking a Catamaran sailboat across the ocean to save the fuel used in airline travel. When she arrived in New York City, hundreds gathered along the shore to welcome her, shouting "Greta, Greta." I am proud to say my son was among them.

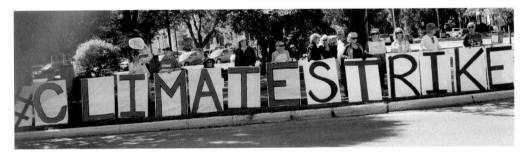

Even older folks joined Greta's climate strike in September 2019. The local climate action committee took part in the climate strike in September 2019. I am proud to say I held a letter.

Since then she has spoken to the Pope, and *sparred with the President of the United States.* (2) She does not represent any political party or advocacy group. However, she has had a major impact.

Greta is not alone. College and high school students are forming groups to write letters to their representatives, strike for climate action, and make changes in their dorms and dining halls.

One such group is the *Sunrise Movement.* (3) Another is the Slow Food Group. (4)

The way is clear. Something must be done. *The United Nations' Scientific Panel on Climate Change warns* that "it will be impossible to keep worldwide temperatures at safe levels unless humans change the way they produce food and use land." (5)

We can make a difference

Hopefully some of the changes outlined in the preceding chapters of this book will be a starting point for each of us to initiate change. If enough of us make changes, it will make a "world" of difference. To highlight some ideas:

- Encourage any farmers you know, Cooperative Extension Agents and Future Farmers of America groups to use sustainable farming methods
- Never buy pesticides and sign petitions for their elimination
- Start or continue a backyard garden, community garden, container garden or hydroponic garden
- Buy close to home - from local growers, CSAs and farmer's markets
- Eliminate or at least cut down the red meat in your diet
- Avoid bacon, ham and other processed meat
- Avoid antibiotic-raised poultry
- Eat low-mercury fish often
- Buy a water filter instead of bottled water
- Plant a tree or trees, especially fruit trees
- Emphasize nutrient-dense foods
- Make vegetables and fruits the main part of your plate
- Use whole-grain breads and pastas
- Cook nutritious brown rice or wild rice (instead of white rice) as an occasional side dish
- Drink soda only as a special treat
- Buy organic if at all possible
- Avoid processed foods and added chemicals and dyes
- Use liquid fats such as canola oil and olive oil
- Cut down on sugar
- Cut down on salty foods
- Limit your open-refrigerator time

- Use cloth bags for shopping
- Avoid paper and plastic products
- Use leftovers
- Turn off the heat cycle in your dishwasher
- Recycle as much as possible
- Support your local recycling center

Some non-food related suggestions:

- Buy solar panels or become part of a solar collective
- Use solar energy to dry your clothes on an outdoor line
- Insulate your house
- Caulk leaks in windows
- Turn down the heat in cold weather
- Use air conditioning sparingly
- Replace light bulbs with LED bulbs
- Turn off lights you are not using
- Turn off computers, and other equipment when you are not using it
- Encourage your community to become a Climate Smart Community
- Buy a hybrid or electric car
- Vote for candidates who support climate change legislation

According to the book, *Drawdown: the most Comprehensive Plan ever Proposed to Reverse Global Warming* edited by Paul Hawken, food-related solutions are some of the least expensive and most effective solutions to the huge climate change problem we are facing. (6) Of course, energy sources and types of transportation are also very important, but more costly solutions.

Do not give up hope. There is much that we can do.

I don't want to preach. I have found some of these things difficult. Make changes a little at a time. I have not always followed these guidelines, but I do try. I only ask you to try as well.

Become part of the solution.

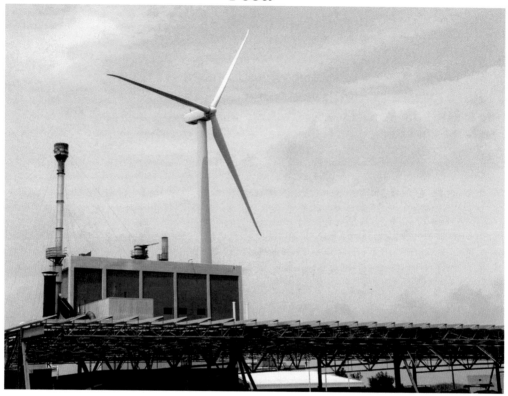

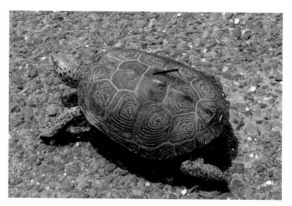

Within sight of the Atlantic City,
New Jersey casinos, Atlantic County has installed a series of windmills that
take advantage of wind currents from the Atlantic Ocean. The area shading
the parking lot is filled with solar panels. They even provide protection for
endangered tortoises which are allowed to roam free.

Sally West Carman

Food

End Notes

Chapter one

1. https://scripps.ucsd.edu/news/carbon-dioxide-levels-hit-record-peak-may

2. https://en.wikipedia.org/wiki/Ice_core

3. Tickell, Josh, *Kiss the Ground,* Simon and Schuster, Inc., 2017, p.14.

4. https://www.coolearth.org/2018/10/ipcc-report-2/

5. Mann, Michael E. and Kump, Lee R. "Dire Predictions, Understanding Climate change" Penguin Random House, 2015, p. 18.

6. *A global multiproxy database for temperature reconstructions of the Common Era, Scientific Data volume 4, Article number: 170088,* 2017, https://www.nature.com/articles/sdata201788.
and, *A global multiproxy database for temperature reconstructions of the Common Era, Scientific Data volume 4, Article number: 170088,* 2017, https://www.nature.com/articles/sdata201788.

7. Amadeo, Kimberly, *Hurricane Sandy Facts, Damage and Economic Impact*, The Balance, September 22, 2018. https://www.thebalance.com/hurricane-sandy-damage-facts-3305501

8. https://www.britannica.com/event/Hurricane-Katrina

9.   https://www.nhc.noaa.gov/data/tcr/AL092017_Harvey.
     pdf

10. https://www.nbcnews.com/news/us-news/rising-
     seas-threaten-norfolk-naval-shipyard-raising-fears-
     catastrophic-damage-n937396

11. Permafrost in a Warming World, Weather Underground,
     https://www.wundergournd.com/resources/climate/
     melting_permafrost.

12. Pero, James, Daily Mail.com, April 2, 2019. https://
     dailymail.co.uk/scientech/article-687415/Melting-
     permafrost.

13. Alaska Public Lands, Permafrost,
     https://www.alaskacenters.gov/explore/attractions/
     permafrost
     and Irving, Michael, New Atlas. Com, April 20th, 2018,
     https://newatlas.com/pleistocene-park-mammoth-
     ecosystem/54257/

14. *The Grapes of Wrath,* https://en.wikipedia.org/wiki/The_
     Grapes_of_Wrath

15. Tickell, Josh, *Kiss the Ground,* Simon and Schuster, Inc.,
     2017, p. 106. And "The global water crisis" *The Week,*
     March 2, 2018, p. 11.

16. https://www.lundberg.com/

17. http://www.greyrockfarmcsa.com/

18. Florida Department of Environmental Protection, https://
     floridadep.gov/fgs/sinkholes.

19. Earthquakes in Oklahoma, date provided by the U.S.
     Geological Survey, http://earthquakes.ok.gov/what-we-
     know/

20. Wernick, Alan, *Climate change will accelerate extreme weather events in the coming years*, PRI, February 18, 2018. https://www.pri.org/stories/2018-02-18/climate-change-will-accelerate-extreme-weather-events-coming-years

21. Amanpour, Christiane, *Interview of Retired Rear Admiral of the Navy, David Titley,* PBS, March 7, 2019. https://www.thirteen.org/programs/amanpour-co/david-titley-climate-change-national-security-risk-fxjufl/; also on: https://slate.com/technology/2014/04/david-titley-climate-change-war-an-interview-with-the-retired-rear-admiral-of-the-navy.html

22. Aronson, Emma L. and and Steven D. Allison, *Meta-Analysis of Environmental Impacts on Nitrous Oxide Release in Response to N Amendment,* https://www.ncbi.nlm.nih.gov/pmc/articles/PMC3408851/

23. Lappé, Frances Moore and Anna Lappé, *Hope's Edge*, Jeremy P. Tarcher/Penguin Group, 2003, p. 8.

Also see:

Johnson, Ian, *Climate change: Nearly 700 'natural thermometers' demonstrate the world is warmer than its ever been, The Independent,* July 12, 2017. https://www.independent.co.uk/environment/climate-change-natural-thermometers-global-warming-world-temperatures-rising-warmest-ever-hockey-a7837881.html

Ibid., 31 scientific bodies tell US Congress: Climate change is real, The Independent, June 28, 2016. https://www.independent.co.uk/environment/climate-change-is-real-experts-tell-us-congress-global-warming-a7107531.html

Sims, Alexandra, *Climate change breakthrough as Iceland turns carbon dioxide into stone, The Independent,* June 9,

2016. https://www.independent.co.uk/news/world/europe/
climate-change-breakthrough-as-iceland-turns-carbon-
dioxide-into-snow-a7073691.html
Harmon, Dwayne, *High Arctic temperatures break records,
Newburgh Gazette,* March 2, 2018. http://newburghgazette.
com/2018/03/02/high-arctic-temperatures-break-records/

Chapter two

1. Carson, Rachel, *Silent Spring,* Houghton Mifflin Company,
    1962.

2. Tickell, Josh, *Kiss the Ground,* Simon and Schuster, Inc.,
    2017, pp. 50-51

3. *Ibid.,* 52.

4. Zhang Luoping,aIemaan Ranaa, Rachel M.Shaffer,
    EmanuelaTaiolic, LianneSheppard, *Exposure to glyphosate-
    based herbicides and risk for non-Hodgkin lymphoma: A meta-
    analysis and supporting evidence,* Science Direct, Volume
    781, July–September 2019, pages 186-206.

5. Tickell, p. 69.

6. https://www.usgs.gov/science-explorer-results?es=atrazine

7. Center for the Health Assessment of Mothers and Children,
    a joint project with the University of Califormia at Berkeley).
    https://www.niehs.nih.gov/research/supported/cohort/
    resources/cohort755393.cfm andhttps://biomonitoring.
    ca.gov/projects/center-health-assessment-mothers-and-
    children-salinas-chamacos.

8. https://en.wikipedia.org/wiki/Genetically_modified_organism

9. O'Neill, Maggie, *Does Cheerios Cause Cancer? Everything You
    Need to Know About Glyphosate,* June 13, 2019. https://

www.health.com/nutrition/cheerios-cancer

10. Sustainable Pulse, *Bob's Red Mill Faces Class Action Lawsuit over Glyphosate Weedkiller Contamination,* September 5, 2018. https://sustainablepulse.com/2018/09/05/bobs-red-mill-faces-class-action-lawsuit-over-glyphosate-weedkiller-contamination/#.XE4gdyx7ncs

11. Van Hoesen, Shannon, EWG, *World Health Organization Labels Glyphosate Probable Carcinogen,* March 20, 2015. https://www.ewg.org/release/world-health-organization-labels-glyphosate-probable-carcinogen

12. Gonzales, Richard, *California Jury Awards $2 Billion To Couple In Roundup Weed Killer Cancer, NPR.org, May 13, 2019.* "Alva and Alberta Pilliod of Livermore, Calif., contracted non-Hodgkin's lymphoma because of their use of the glyphosate-based herbicide." https://www.npr.org/2019/05/13/723056453/california-jury-awards-2-billion-to-couple-in-roundup-weed-killer-cancer-trial

13. Consumer Safety, https://www.consumersafety.org/legal/roundup-lawsuit/
Monsanto faces 11,200+ Roundup lawsuits, including one in which the plaintiff received a jury award of $78.5 million in compensatory and punitive damages.

14. Little, Amanda, *The Fate of Food,* Harmony Books, 2019, p. 89 and Taylor, Alan, *Bhopal: The World's Worst Industrial Disaster, 30 Years Later,* "The Atlantic", Dec 2, 2014.

15. Tickell, p. 63.

16. Chiller, Tom, Center for Disease Control and Prevention. https://www.11alive.com/article/news/deadly-fungus-infection-spreads-in-hospitals/85-1742ce57-7202-463a-a923-5d3347e7b9a9

17. Friends of the Earth Newsletter, *Food retailers fail to protect bees from toxic pesticides,* Vol. 48, No. 1, Spring 2018, p. 2.

18. Sánchez-Bayoa, Francisco and Kris A.G.Wyckhuys, *Worldwide decline of the entomofauna: A review of its drivers,* Biological Conservation, Volume 232, April 2019, Pages 8-27, https://www.sciencedirect.com/science/article/pii/S0006320718313636

19. Bates, Theunis, Managing editor, *The Week,* February 23, 2019.

20. National Geographic for kids, *Lady bug,* https://kids.nationalgeographic.com/animals/ladybug/#ladybug-daisy.jpg

21. https://www.discoverlife.org/

22. National Ocean Service, https://oceanservice.noaa.gov/facts/redtide.html

23. Zerkel, Eric, The Weather Channel, *Toledo, Ohio Water Supply Contaminated by Algae From Lake Erie,* August 03, 2014. https://weather.com/news/news/toledo-ohio-water-algae-lake-erie-20140802

24. https://www.healthline.com/health/is-red-tide-harmful-to-humans.

Chapter three

1. Tickell, p. 26.

2. https://www.investopedia.com/articles/company-insights/090216/top-5-companies-owned-cargill.asp

3. Pollan, Michael, *Omnivore's Dilemma,* pp. 52-53.

4. Ohlson, Kristin, *The soil will save us,* p. 80.

5. https://smallfarms.cornell.edu/2015/10/reducing-tillage/

6. Barth, Brian, *Permaculture: You've Heard of It, But What the Heck Is It?* April 19, 2016. *https*://modernfarmer. com/2016/04/permaculture/ and http://www.neverendingfood.org/b-what-permaculture/

6. Sustainable Agriculture Research and Education, *Types of Cover Crops*, University of Maryland, College Park, MD. https://www.sare.org/Learning-Center/Books/Building-Soils-for-Better-Crops-3rd-Edition/Text-Version/Cover-Crops/Types-of-Cover-Crops

7. *Cattle Grazing Cover Crops in Southern Minnesota,* USDA, https://www.nrcs.usda.gov/wps/portal/nrcs/ mn/newsroom/features/7060c5de-b5f5-44fe-9e1d-35c9271d0a4a/ and https://nrcs.maps.arcgis.com/apps/ Cascade/index.html?appid=b5ea142e56e14ffb8f7322cc2b2 1c720

8. Barber, Dan, *The Third Plate*, Penguin Books, 2013, pp. 71-72.

9. *Ibid.*, p. 12-13.

10.. *Friends of the Earth News*, Vol 48, no. 1, Spring 2018, p. 2. https://foe.org/news/

Chapter four

1. Edwards, Chris, Director of Policy Studies, *Downsizing the Federal Government*, Cato Institute. www.cato.downsizinggovenment.org

2. https://www.openthebooks.com/

3. https://www.washingtonpost.com/

4. Johnson, Marie, *The land of milk and money: Dairy farmers cope with chronically low milk prices, uncertain futures*, Agweek, July 4 2018. https://www.agweek.com/business/agriculture/4468598-land-milk-and-money-dairy-farmers-cope-chronically-low-milk-prices

Chapter five

1. Lappé, Frances Moore and Anna Lappé, *Hope's Edge*, Jeremy P. Tarcher/Penguin Group, 2003, p. 237, 287.

2. The Daily Beast, *10 Facts About Mad Cow Diseases*, April 25, 2014. https://www.thedailybeast.com/10-facts-about-mad-cow-diseases

3. Wikipedia, *Food libel laws*, https://en.wikipedia.org/wiki/Food_libel_laws.

4. Wein, Dr. Harrison, *Risk in Red Meat?* National Institute of Health, March 26, 2012. https://www.nih.gov/news-events/nih-research-matters/risk-red-meat

5. *Harvard Researchers: Red meat consumption tied to early death.* Harvard Health Letter, Vol. 44, Number 11, September 2019.

6. NHS, *Red meat and the risk of bowel cancer* https://www.nhs.uk/live-well/eat-well/red-meat-and-the-risk-of-bowel-cancer/

7. The Scientific Advisory Committee on Nutrition recommendations on iron and health, and consumption of red and processed meat, February 25, 2011.

8. *Harvard Women's Health Watch*, September 2019, p. 3.

9. Oppenlander, Dr. Richard A., *Comfortably Unaware*, Beaufort Books, New York, 2012, p. 54, 84, 108.

10. https://jamanetwork.com/journals/jamainternalmedicine/article-abstract/2767106?widget=personalizedcontent&previousarticle=2748453

11. How much water does it take to make a hamburger, https://water.usgs.gov/edu

Also see:
Moser, Whet, *Horse Meat: Good Enough for the Mafia and the Greatest Generation, But Not For Picky Non-Pagan Modern Consumers,* Chicago Magazine, February 1, 2013. https://www.chicagomag.com/Chicago-Magazine/The-312/February-2013/Horse-Meat-Good-Enough-for-the-Mafia-and-the-Greatest-Generation-But-Not-For-Picky-Non-Pagan-Modern-Consumers/

Chapter six

1. Scientific American, *How Does Mercury Get Into Fish?* https://www.scientificamerican.com/article/how-does-mercury-get-into/

2. Greenberg, Paul, *American Catch*, Penguin Books, NYC, NY, 2014, p. 178.

3. National Institute of Health, *Omega 3 Fatty acids.* https://ods.od.nih.gov/factsheets/Omega3FattyAcids-HealthProfessional/

4. Brown, Dr. Mary Jane, *Should You Avoid Fish Because of Mercury?* Healthline, September 14, 2016. https://www.healthline.com/nutrition/mercury-content-of-fish

5. American Heart Association, *Saturated Fat*, June 1, 2015.

https://www.heart.org/en/healthy-living/healthy-eating/eat-smart/fats/saturated-fats

6. Webmd, *What You Need to Know about Mercury in Fish and Shellfish,*
    https://www.webmd.com/diet/mercury-in-fish#1

7. Oregon State University, *Essential Fatty Acids,* 2019. https://lpi.oregonstate.edu/mic/other-nutrients/essential-fatty-acids

8. Wikipedia, *Omega-6 fatty acid*
    https://en.wikipedia.org/wiki/Omega-6_fatty_acid

Chapter seven

1. Balogh, James, *The Human Element,* documentary, 2018.

2. Kusnetz, Nicholas, *Rising seas threaten Norfolk Naval Shipyard, raising fears of 'catastrophic damage',* NBCNews.com and InsideClimate News, Nov. 2018. https://www.nbcnews.com/news/us-news/rising-seas-threaten-norfolk-naval-shipyard-raising-fears-catastrophic-damage-n937396

3. https://insideclimatenews.org/news/18012019/military-bases-climate-change-risks-wildfires-flooding-defense-department-report-congress

4. Bodiner, Chris, *The Science Behind Florida's Sinkhole Epidemic,* Smithsonian Magazine, May 24, 2018. https://www.smithsonianmag.com/science-nature/science-behind-floridas-sinkhole-epidemic-180969158/

5. Calma, Justin, *MTA floods NYC subway entrance because 'climate change is real',* November 21, 2019. https://www.theverge.com/2019/11/21/20976248/mta-floods-test-nyc-subway-climate-change-equipment-flex-gate

6. Lallanilla, Marc, *Facts About Fracking,* February 10, 2018,

https://www.livescience.com/34464-what-is-fracking.html.

7.   Brodwin, Erin, *Parts of Oklahoma now have the same earthquake risk as California — and a new study found a scarily direct link to fracking*, Business Insider, February 2, 2018, https://www.businessinsider.com/earthquakes-fracking-oklahoma-research-2018-2

8.   Environmental Protection Agency, *Nutrient Pollution: The Sources and Solutions: Agriculture* https://www.epa.gov/nutrientpollution/sources-and-solutions-agriculture

9.   https://www.sciencedaily.com/releases/2008/01/080130092108.htm

Chapter eight

1.   Wikipedia, *Johnny Appleseed.*
      https://en.wikipedia.org/wiki/Johnny_Appleseed

2.   Pollan, Michael, *The Botany of Desire:A Plant's Eye View of the World*, Random House, 2002.
      https://michaelpollan.com/wp-content/uploads/2010/06/botany_of_desire_excerpt.pdf

3.   Friends of the Earth, *Toxic Secret: Pesticides uncovered in store brand cereal, beans, produce,* https://foe.org/food-testing-results/.

4.   Yoshioka, Wayne, *Hawai'i Becomes First State to Ban Neurotoxin, Chlorpyrifos,* Hawaii Public Radio, June 13, 2018.
      https://www.hawaiipublicradio.org/post/hawaii-becomes-first-state-ban-neurotoxin-chlorpyrifos

5.   Callahan, Catherine, et. al., *Chlorpyrifos Exposure and Respiratory Health among Adolescent Agricultural Workers,* The International Journal of Environmental Research and

Public Health, December 11, 2014.

6. National Resource Defense Council (NRDC), *Nature's Voice,* Summer 2020.

7. Environmental Health, Maternal and Reproductive Health, *Prenatal Exposure to Insecticide Linked to Alterations in Brain Structure and Cognition,* April 30, 2012. https://www.mailman.columbia.edu/public-health-now/ news/prenatal-exposure-insecticide-chlorpyrifos-linked-alterations-brain-structure

8. Hughes, Roland, *Amazon fires: What's the latest in Brazil?* BBC News, October 12, 2019, https://www.bbc.com/news/ world-latin-america-49971563.

9. https://www.fastcompany.com/2681925/a-simple-elegant-stove-to-make-cooking-safer-in-africa and https://envirofit.org/ products/east-africa/

10. Arango, Tim, Jose A. Del Real and Ivan Penn, NYTimes, *5 Lessons We Learned From the California Wildfires,* Nov. 4, 2019, https://www.nytimes.com/2019/11/04/us/fires-california.html.

Chapter nine

1. https://en.wikipedia.org/wiki/Living_with_the_Land

2. Steven McFadden, Community Agriculture Author, Mother Earth News, https://www.motherearthnews.com/ biographies/steven-mcfadden-community-supported-agriculture-author

3.. Biodynamic Association, *Community Supported Agriculture: An Introduction to CSA,* East Troy, WI. https://www. biodynamics.com/content/community-supported-agriculture-introduction-csa

4. Brafman, Isabella and Ed Yowell, *The "Slow" Green New Deal*, Slow Food USA, Feb. 24, 2019. https://www.slowfoodusa.org/blog-post/the-slow-green-new-deal

5. https://www.washingtonpost.com/business/2018/12/11/congresss-billion-farm-bill-is-out-heres-whats-it/?noredirect=on&utm_term=.d57cf1c44b3f

Chapter ten

1. Liebman, Bonnie, *Nutrition Action,* Center for Science in the Public Interest, March 11, 2019. https://www.nutritionaction.com/daily/what-to-eat/the-grandparents-diet/

2. Loria, Kevin, *Leavy Greens Safety Guide, Consumer Reports*, March 2020, pp. 26- 37.

3. Bjarnadottir, Adda MS, LN, *Tomatoes 101: Nutrition Facts and Health Benefits, Healthline*, Healthline, March 25, 2019. https://www.healthline.com/nutrition/foods/tomatoes

4. https://www.researchgate.net/scientific-contributions/2139136868_Joshua_W_Miller

5. "The Essential Nutrient You May Be Missing", *On Health*, newsletter by Consumer Reports, Jun3 2019. CR.org/missingnutrients

6. Van Horn Linda , Marilyn Cornelis, Dr. John Wilkins, Dr. Hongyan Ning, Mercedes Carnethon, Dr. Philip Greenland, Lihui Zhao and Dr. Donald Lloyd-Jones, Northwestern University Study, *Higher egg and cholesterol consumption hikes heart disease and early death risk,* Science Daily, March 15, 2019.

https://www.sciencedaily.com/releases/2019/03/190315110858.htm
And https://www.healthline.com/nutrition/how-many-eggs-should-you-eat

7. https://news.globallandscapesforum.org/39372/thought-for-food-walter-willett-on-diet-for-personal-and-planetary-health/

8. McColloch, Marsha, MS RD, *Nutritional benefits of walnuts,* Healthline, July 9, 2018. https://www.healthline.com/nutrition/benefits-of-walnuts#section4

9. *Circulation,* Volume 139, issue 8, February 9, 2019, as reported in *Health Wire,* a newsletter of Consumer Reports, June 2019. https://www.ahajournals.org/toc/circ/139/8

10. Center for Science in the Public Interest, Library. https://cspinet.org/library

11. Willett, Walter, *What's New in Eat, Drink, and Be Healthy,* 2017, https://www.hsph.harvard.edu/nutritionsource/2017/10/15/eat-drink-and-be-healthy-willett/

12. https://www.webmd.com/healthy-aging/omega-3-fatty-acids-fact-sheet#1

13. Why is celery powder so controversial? https://newfoodeconomy.org/organic-celery-powder-nosb-vote/

14. de Salcedo, Anastacia Marx, *Combat Ready Kitchen,* Penguin Random House, 2015, pp. 225-228.

15. https://www.nhlbi.nih.gov/health/educational/wecan/downloads/tip-sugar-in-drinks.pdf

16. *Artificial sweeteners and other sugar substitutes,* https://www.mayoclinic.org/healthy-lifestyle/nutrition-and-healthy-

eating/in-depth/artificial-sweeteners/art-20046936

17. *What is Stevia,* https://www.medicalnewstoday.com/articles/287251#what_is_stevia

18. https://www.medicalnewstoday.com/articles/324997#antibacterial

19. *Everything you need to know about molasses* https://www.medicalnewstoday.com/articles/318719#nutrition

20. *Are Plant Milks Good for You?* https://www.consumerreports.org/plant-milk/are-plant-milks-more-healthful-than-cows-milk/

21. https://www.webmd.com/parenting/baby/news/20080711/baby-milk-recommendations-changed

22. Hirsch, Jessie, *Arsenic and Lead Are in Your Fruit Juice: What You Need to Know*, Consumer Reports, January 30, 2019. https://www.consumerreports.org/food-safety/arsenic-and-lead-are-in-your-fruit-juice-what-you-need-to-know/

23. Amidor, Tony, *5 Surprising Health Benefits of Beer*, U.S. News and World Report, September 30, 2016. https://health.usnews.com/health-news/blogs/eat-run/articles/2016-12-30/5-surprising-health-benefits-of-beer

24. Mayo Clinic staff, *Caffeine content for coffee, tea, soda and more*, Mayo Clinic, April 14, 2017. https://www.mayoclinic.org/healthy-lifestyle/nutrition-and-healthy-eating/in-depth/caffeine/art-20049372

25. Pennington, Jean A. T. and Judith Spungen, Bowes and Church Food Values of Portions Commonly Used, 19th edition, Lippincott, Williams and Wilkins, 2010, pp. 284-286.

26. Tea: A cup of good health? Harvard Men's Health Watch, August, 2014. https://www.health.harvard.edu/press_releases/health-benefits-linked-to-drinking-tea

27. Carroll, Aaron E., Health Benefits of Tea? Here's What the Evidence Says, New York Times, August 15, 2015. https://www.nytimes.com/2015/10/06/upshot/what-the-evidence-tells-us-about-tea.html

28 https://www.consumerreports.org/bottled-water/should-we-break-our-bottled-water-habit/

29. https://www.consumerreports.org/water-quality/find-out-whats-in-your-bottled-water-water-quality-reports/ and https://www.consumerreports.org/bottled-water/should-we-break-our-bottled-water-habit/

30. https://www.foodandwaterwatch.org/about/live-healthy/tap-water-vs-bottled-water

31. https://www.nytimes.com/2019/03/29/business/poland-spring-water.html

32. https://www.bloomberg.com/news/articles/2019-11-01/how-coke-pepsi-and-nestle-plan-to-profit-from-your-tap-water

33. Centers for Disease Control and Prevention, *About Antibiotic Resistance*, September 10, 2018. https://www.cdc.gov/drugresistance/about.html

34. https://www.pbs.org/wgbh/pages/frontline/shows/meat/safe/overview.html

35. Williams, Holly, *A bigger killer than cancer,* April 21, 2019. https://www.cbsnews.com/news/could-antibiotic-resistant-

superbugs-become-a-bigger-killer-than-cancer-60-minutes-2019-04-21/

36. https://www.fda.gov/consumers/consumer-updates/antibacterial-soap-you-can-skip-it-use-plain-soap-and-water

37. Stromberg, Joseph, Five Reasons Why You Should Probably Stop Using Antibacterial Soap, January 3, 2014, https://www.smithsonianmag.com/science-nature/five-reasons-why-you-should-probably-stop-using-antibacterial-soap-180948078/

35. Centers for Disease Control and Prevention, *Triclosan Factsheet*, April 7, 2017.   https://www.cdc.gov/biomonitoring/Triclosan_FactSheet.html

Chapter eleven

1. When Going Organic Matters Most for You, Cleveland Clinic, July 10, 2014, https://health.clevelandclinic.org/when-going-organic-matters-most-for-you/

2. Easy life for seniors, 15 Things You Should Never Buy From the Supermarket, September 24, 2018. https://easyseniorslife.com/curiosities/15-things-you-should-never-buy-from-the-supermarket/14/

3. https://www.hungryharvest.net/

4. https://www.washingtonpost.com/sf/brand-connect/sub-zero/solving-the-problem-of-food-waste/

5. https://www.dentistryiq.com/dental-hygiene/student-hygiene/article/16366229/does-ph-matter-the-role-of-water-in-dental-patients-diets

6. Schecter, Arnold, et. al., *Bisphenol A (BPA) in U.S. Food*, https://pubs.acs.org/doi/full/10.1021/es102785d, November 1, 2010.

7. CBSNews.com as reported in *The Week, March 29, 2019.*

8. *https://health.clevelandclinic.org/5-reasons-fruit-veggies-csa-farms-different/*

9. *https://www.dentistryiq.com/dental-hygiene/student-hygiene/article/16366229/does-ph-matter-the-role-of-water-in-dental-patients-diets : "The cost for bottled water compared to tap water was steep because the price of a gallon of bottled water was 10,000 times that for tap water"*

Chapter thirteen

1. Chlorofluorcarbons (CFCs), https://www.esrl.noaa.gov/gmd/hats/publictn/elkins/cfcs.html

2. Hawkin, Paul, *Drawdown: the most Comprehensive Plan ever Proposed to Reverse Global Warming*, pp. 224-225.

3. cnygreenbucketproject.org

4, https://en.wikipedia.org/wiki/Pulp_mill

5. https://www.terracycle.com/en-US/collection-programs and https://www.terracycle.com/en-US/brigades

6. Kwan, Nicole, *Rethinking Recycling*, Subaru Drive Magazine, Spring/Summer 2019, p. 9.

Chapter fourteen

1. Little, Amanda, *The Fate of Food,* Harmony Books, 2019, pp 98-102..

2. *Ibid*, pp. 103-104..

3. *Ibid*. p.130.

4. *Ibid*, pp. 127-128..

5. *Ibid*, pp. 129-131.

6. Hawkin, Paul, *Drawdown: the most Comprehensive Plan ever Proposed to Reverse Global Warming*, pp. 224-225.

7. Pritchard, Charles, Giant greenhouse gets going and growing, *Rome Sentinel*, January 8, 2020,https://romesentinel.com/stories/giant-greenhouse-gets-going-and-growing,89740

8. https://www.syracuse.com/coronavirus/2020/05/green-empire-farms-outbreak-madison-county-tests-150-more-farmworkers-for-coronavirus.html

9. Little, pp.249-250.

10. *Ibid.*, pp. 247-248.

11. Grain, *The Great Climate Robbery,* New Internationalist Publications Ltd., Oxford, U.K., 2016.

12. https://en.wikipedia.org/wiki/Impossible_Foods

13. https://vegnews.com/2019/1/impossible-foods-unveils-impossible-burger-20

14. Little, p. 173.

15. https://www.organicconsumers.org/fww-oca-sue-tyson-for-deceptive-advertising?utm_medium=email&utm_source=engagingnetworks&utm_campaign=OB+630&utm_content=OB+630+Sunday

Food

16. *Healthletter.MayoClinic.com,* April 2020, p. 8.

17. de Salcedo, Anastacia Marx, *Combat Ready Kitchen,* Penguin Random House, 2015, pp. 31

18. Little, pp. 260-261.

19 *Ibid,* p. 266.

20. *Ibid,* p. 168.

21. Mandyck, John M. and Eric B. Schultz, *Food Foolish: the hidden connection between food waste, hunger and climate change,* Carrier Corporation, 2015, p. 35.

22. *Ibid.* p. 49.

23. https://en.wikipedia.org/wiki/Geritol

24. https://maritime-executive.com/article/worlds-first-hydrogen-powered-cruise-ship-scheduled

25. Trauthwein, Greg, *Maritime Propulsion,* December 28, 2017, https://www.maritimepropulsion.com/news/lng-maritime-fuel-the-532486

26. Rifkin, Jeremy, *The Hydrogen Economy: the next great economic revolution,* Penguin Group, New York, 2002, p. 255.

Chapter fifteen

1. Alter, Charlotte, Suyin Haynes and Justin Worland, *The Conscience,* December 23 - 30, 2019, pp. 50-64.

2. Flesonthal, Edward, *Greta Thunberg, Time's Person of the Year, 2019, Time Magazine,* December 23, 2019.

3. https://www.sunrisemovement.org/about

4. https://www.slowfood.com/about-us/our-philosophy/

5. Hawkin, Paul, *Drawdown: the most Comprehensive Plan ever Proposed to Reverse Global Warming*, pp. 224-225.

6. Neuberger, Emma, *Climate change could trigger an international food crisis*, UN panel warns,   https://www.cnbc.com/2019/08/07/un-climate-panel-urges-land-use-changes-to-avert-food-crisis.htm

Food

Sources

I received information and inspiration from members of the Climate Action Sub-committee of the Unitarian Universalist Church of Utica and the following sources:

Barber, Dan, *The Third Plate*, Penguin Books, New York City, New York, 2014.

de Salcedo, Anastacia Marx, *Combat-Ready Kitchen*, Penguin Random House, New York City, New York, 2015.

GRAIN, *The Great Climate Robbery,* New Internationalist Publications Ltd., Oxford, United Kingdom, 2016.

Greenberg, Paul, *American Catch: the Fight for our Local Seafood,* Penguin Books, New York City, New York, 2015.

Hawkins, Paul, editor, *Drawdown: the Most Comprehensive Plan Ever Proposed to Reverse Global Warming,* Penguin Random House, New York City, New York, 2017.

Lappé, Francis Moore, *Diet for a Small Planet*, Ballantine Books, New York City, New York, 1971.

Lappé, Francis Moore and Anna Lappé, *Hope's Edge: The Next Diet for a Small Planet*, Putnam/Penguin Random House, New York City, New York, 2002-2003.

Lappé, Anna, *Diet for a Hot Planet: the Climate Crisis at the End of your Fork and What You Can Do About It,* Bloomsbury, New York, 2010.

Food

Little, Amanda, *Fate of Food*, Harmony Books, New York City, New York, 2019.

McKibben, Bill, *Falter: Has the Human Game Begun to Play Itself Out?* Henry Holt and Company, New York, 2019.

Nestle, Marion, *Food Politics: How the Food Industry Influences Nutrition and Health*, University of California Press, Berkeley - Los Angeles, California, 2013.

Ohlson, Kristin, *The Soil Will Save Us: How Scientists, Farmers, and Foodies Are Healing the Soil to Save the Planet*, Rodale Books, New York City, New York, 2014.

Mann, Michael E. and Lee R. Kump, *Dire Predictions: Understanding Climate Change*, Penguin Random House, New York, New York, 2015.

Mandyck, John M. And Eric B. Schultz, *Food Foolish: the Hidden Connection between Food Waste, Hunger and Climate Change*, Carrier Corporation, 2017.

Montgomery, David R., *Growing a Revolution: Bringing our Soil Back to Live*, W. W. Norton and Company, New York City, New York, 2017.

Oppenlander, Dr. Richard A., *Comfortably Unaware: what we choose to eat is killing us and our planet*, Beaufort Books, New York City, New York, 2012.

Pennington, Jean A. T. and Judith Spungen, *Bowes and Church's Food Values of Portions Commonly Used*, nineteenth edition, Wolters Kluwer/ Lippincott Williams & Wilkins, Philadelphia, PA, 2010.

Pollan, Michael, *In Defense of Food: an Eater's Manifesto*, Penguin Books, New York City, New York, 2008.

Pollan, Michael, *Omnivore's Dilemma: a Natural History of Four Meals,* Penguin Random House, New York City, New York, 2006.

Prescott, Matthew, *Food is the Solution: What to Eat to Save the World,* Flatiron Books, New York City, New York, 2018.

Rifkin, Jeremy, *The Hydrogen Economy: the Next Great Economic Revolution,* Penguin Group, New York City, New York, 2003.

Schlosser, Eric, *Fast Food Nation,* Houghton Mifflin Company, New York City, New York, 2001.

Tickell, Josh, *Kiss the Ground: How the Food You Eat Can Reverse Climate Change, Heal Your Body and Ultimately Save Our World,* Simon and Schuster, Inc., New York City, New York, 2017.

Wagner, Gernot and Martin L. Weitzman, *Climate Shock,* Princeton University Press, Princeton, New Jersey, 2015.

Wong, James, *How to Eat Better: Simple Science to Supercharge Your Nutrition,* Sterling Epicure, New York, 2017.

Food

Index

Symbols

2,4-D 17

A

AeroFarms 156
Agent Orange 17
agriculture 9, 27
algae 20, 91, 161, 162
Alzheimer's Disease 105
Amazon 44, 57
American Catch 48
American Medical Association 44
anaerobic incinerator 148
Adam Andrzejewski 35
antibacterial 90, 91
antibiotics 41, 89, 90, 91
antioxidant 46, 78
astaxanthin 46
atrazine 15

B

James Balogh 50
Bananas 138, 162
Dan Barber 31
Bayer vii
bee 18
beef 17, 40, 41, 42, 43, 44, 45, 57, 77, 79, 83, 90, 159, 160
Bees 18
Beyond Meat 160
biotin 74
Blue River 154, 155
Representative Anthony Brindisi vi
Patrick Brown 159

C

caffeine 87, 88, 97
Camp Fire 9
candida auris 17

Q

quinoa 9

R

Rachel Carson iii
rainforest 44
recycling 12, 96, 99, 148, 149, 150, 151, 152, 153, 170
Red Tide 20, 21
refrigerants 146, 163
reusable bags 100, 153
reusing 12
riboflavin 74
Jeremy Rifkin 164
Robots 154
Roundup 14

S

salmon 46, 47, 48, 75, 162
sand storms 8
saturated fat 43, 45, 77, 80, 87, 159
Scientific Advisory Committee on Nutrition 44
Scripps Institution of Oceanography 5
See and Spray 155
sell by" date 107
Silent Spring iii, 14
Slow Food Group 168
Smithsonian Magazine 51
solar panels 163, 170
steaming rack 106
John Steinbeck 8
Stone Barns Center 31
straws 100, 101, 102
Styrofoam 151
Subaru 151, 152
subsidies 34, 35
Sunrise Movement 168
sustainable 5, 9, 29, 31, 32, 57, 69, 70, 95, 169
Syracuse University iv, 73
Syria 11

T

Terra Cycle 151
The Grapes of Wrath 8
thiamine 74

Sally West Carman

Food

About the author

With a Master of Arts in Nutrition from Syracuse University (1982), Sally West Carman has long had a interest in the nutrient content of food. As early as the 1970s she developed an avid interest in the environment and the impact of humans on the world in which we live. She is deeply concerned about the impact that climate change will have on our children, our grandchildren, extinction of various animals and plants, and socioeconomic disruption.

Sally has held a number of positions. Her last was as Administrator of The Levitt Public Affairs Center at Hamilton College. She is a mother, grandmother and great-grandmother. She is currently enjoying retirement and the opportunity to write. Her hobbies include: reading, sewing, line dancing and gardening.

Made in the USA
Middletown, DE
09 August 2021